**A Feast of Information—**

for people who love to eat but need to know
the calorie count of their meals.
BARBARA KRAUS 1991 CALORIE GUIDE
TO BRAND NAMES AND BASIC FOODS
lists thousands of basic and ready-to-eat foods,
from appetizers to desserts—carry it to the
supermarket, to the restaurant, to the beach, to
the coffee cart, and on trips. Flip through these
fact-filled pages. Mix, match, and keep track of
calories as they add up. But remember, strawberry
shortcake is fattening any way you slice it!

# BARBARA KRAUS
# 1991 CALORIE GUIDE
# TO BRAND NAMES AND
# BASIC FOODS

# Barbara Kraus
# 1991 Calorie
# Guide to
# Brand Names and
# Basic Foods

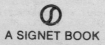

A SIGNET BOOK

For Francine Caruso and Richard Paladino

SIGNET
Published by the Penguin Group
Penguin Books USA Inc., 375 Hudson Street,
New York, New York 10014, U.S.A.
Penguin Books Ltd, 27 Wrights Lane,
London W8 5TZ, England
Penguin Books Australia Ltd, Ringwood,
Victoria, Australia
Penguin Books Canada Ltd, 2801 John Street,
Markham, Ontario, Canada L3R 1B4
Penguin Books (N.Z.) Ltd, 182-190 Wairau Road,
Auckland 10, New Zealand

Penguin Books Ltd, Registered Offices:
Harmondsworth, Middlesex, England

First published by Signet, an imprint of New American Library, a
division of Penguin Books USA Inc.

First Printing, January, 1991
10  9  8  7  6  5  4  3  2  1

# *Foreword*

The composition of the foods we eat is not static: it changes from time to time. In the case of *brand-name* products, manufacturers alter their recipes to reflect the availability of ingredients, advances in technology, or improvements in formulae. Each year new products appear on the market and some old ones are discontinued.

On the other hand, information on *basic foods* such as meats, vegetables, and fruits may also change as a result of the development of better analytical methods, different growing conditions, or new marketing practices. These changes, however, are usually relatively small as compared with those in manufactured products.

Some differences may be found between the values in this book and those appearing on the product labels. This is usually due to the fact that the Food and Drug Administration permits manufacturers to round the figures reported on labels. The data in this book are reported as calculated without rounding. If large differences between the two sets of values are noted, they may be due to changes in product formulae, and in those cases the label data should be used.

For all these reasons, a book of calorie or nutritive values of foods must be kept up to date by a periodic reviewing and revision of the data presented.

Therefore, this handy calorie counter will provide each year the most current and accurate estimates available. Generous use of this little book will help you and your family to select the right foods and the proper number of calories each member requires to gain, lose, or maintain healthy and attractive weight.

*Barbara Kraus*

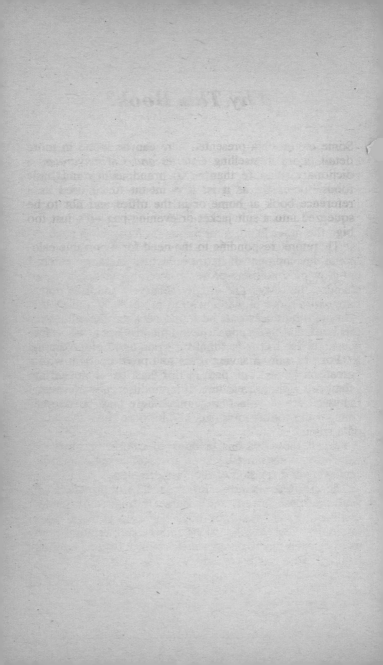

# Why This Book?

Some of the data presented here can be found in more detail in my bestselling *Calories and Carbohydrates,* a dictionary of more than 8,000 brand names and basic foods. Complete as it is, it is meant to be used as a reference book at home or in the office and not to be squeezed into a suit jacket or evening bag—it's just too big.

Therefore, responding to the need for a portable calorie guide, and one which can reflect food changes often, I have written this smaller and handier version. The selection of material and the additional new entries provide readers with pertinent data on thousands of products that they would prepare at home to take to work, eat in a restaurant or luncheonette, nibble on from the coffee cart, take to the beach, buy in the candy store, et cetera.

For the sake of saving space and providing you with a greater selection of products, I had to make certain compromises: whereas in the giant book there are several physical descriptions of a product, here there is but one.

# For Beginners Only

The language of dieting is no more difficult to learn than any other new subject; in many respects, it's much easier, particularly if you restrict your education to clearly defined goals.

For you who never before had the need or the interest in a lesson in weight control, I offer the following elementary introduction, applicable to any diet, self-initiated or suggested by your doctor, nutritionist, or dietician.

### A Calorie

An analysis of foods in terms of calories is most often the chosen method to describe the relative energy yielded by foods.

A calorie is a shorthand way to summarize the units of energy contained in any foodstuff or alcoholic beverage, similar to the way a thermometer indicates heat. One pound of fat is equal to 3,500 calories. Add this number of calories to those you need to balance your energy requirements and you will gain one pound; subtract it and you will lose a pound.

### Other Nutrients

Carbohydrates—which include sugars, starches, and acids—are only one of several chemical compounds in foods that yield calories. Proteins, found mainly in beef, poultry, and fish; fats, found in oils, butter, marbling of meat, and poultry skin; and alcohol, found in some beverages, also contribute calories. Except for alcohol, most foods contain at least some of these nutrients.

The amount of carbohydrates varies from zero in meats and a trace in alcohol to a heavy concentration in sugar, syrups, some fruits, grains, and root vegetables.

As of this date, the most respected nutritional researchers insist that some carbohydrates are necessary every day for maintaining good health. The amount to be included is an individual matter, and in any drastic effort to change your eating patterns, be sure to consult your doctor first.

Now, on how to use this new language.

To begin with, you use this book like a dictionary. If your plan is to cut down on calories, the easiest way to do so is to consult the portable calorie counter and keep an accurate count of your total intake of food and beverages for a period of seven days. If you have not gained or lost weight during that week, divide that number by seven and you'll have your maintenance diet expressed in calories. To lose weight, you must reduce your daily or weekly intake of calories below this maintenance level. (To gain, increase the intake.)

Keeping in mind that you want to stay healthy and eat well-balanced meals (which include the basic food groups: milk or milk products; meat, poultry, or fish; vegetables and fruits; and whole grain or enriched breads or cereals, as well as some fats or oils), you then start to cut down on your portion in order to reduce your intake of calories. There are many imaginative ways to diet without total withdrawal from one's favorite foods.

Once you know and don't have to guess what calories are in your foods, you can relax and enjoy them. It could turn out that dieting isn't so bad after all.

## ABBREVIATIONS AND SYMBOLS

* = prepared as package directs[1]
< = less than
& = and
" = inch
canned = bottles or jars as well as cans
dia. = diameter
fl. = fluid
liq. = liquid
lb. = pound
med. = medium

oz. = ounce
pkg. = package
pt. = pint
qt. = quart
sq. = square
T. = tablespoon
Tr. = trace
tsp. = teaspoon
wt. = weight

Italics or name in parentheses = registered trademark, ®. All data not identified by company or trademark are based on material obtained from the United States Department of Agriculture or Health, Education and Welfare/Food and Agriculture Organization.

## EQUIVALENTS

*By Weight*
1 pound = 16 ounces
1 ounce = 28.35 grams
3.52 ounces = 100 grams

*By Volume*
1 quart = 4 cups
1 cup = 8 fluid ounces
1 cup = ½ pint
1 cup = 16 tablespoons
2 tablespoons = 1 fluid ounce
1 tablespoon = 3 teaspoons
1 pound butter = 4 sticks or 2 cups

[1]If the package directions call for whole or skim milk, the data given here are for whole milk unless otherwise stated.

# A

| Food and Description | Measure or Quantity | Calories |
|---|---|---|
| **ABALONE,** canned | 4 oz. | 91 |
| ***AC'CENT*** | ¼ tsp. | 3 |
| **AGNOLETTI,** frozen (Buitoni): | | |
| Cheese filled | 2-oz. serving | 196 |
| Meat filled | 2-oz. serving | 206 |
| **ALBACORE,** raw, meat only | 4 oz. | 201 |
| **ALLSPICE** (French's) | 1 tsp. | 6 |
| **ALMOND:** | | |
| In shell | 10 nuts | 60 |
| Shelled, raw, natural, with skins | 1 oz. | 170 |
| Roasted, dry (Planters) | 1 oz. | 170 |
| Roasted, honey (Eagle) | 1 oz. | 150 |
| Roasted, oil (Tom's) | 1 oz. | 180 |
| **ALMOND EXTRACT** (Durkee) pure | 1 tsp. | 13 |
| ***ALPHA-BITS,*** cereal (Post) | 1 cup (1 oz.) | 110 |
| ***AMARETTO DI SARONNO*** | 1 fl. oz. | 83 |
| **ANCHOVY, PICKLED,** canned, flat or rolled, not heavily salted, drained (Granadaisa) | 2-oz. can | 80 |
| **ANISE EXTRACT** (Durkee) imitation | 1 tsp. | 16 |
| **ANISETTE:** | | |
| (DeKuyper) | 1 fl. oz. | 95 |
| (Mr. Boston) | 1 fl. oz. | 88 |
| **APPLE:** | | |
| Fresh, with skin | 2½″ dia. | 61 |
| Fresh, without skin | 2½″ dia. | 53 |
| Canned: | | |
| (Comstock): | | |
| Rings, drained | 1 ring | 30 |
| Sliced | ⅙ of 21-oz. can | 45 |
| (White House): | | |
| Rings | 1 ring | 11 |
| Sliced | ½ cup (4 oz.) | 54 |
| Dried: | | |
| (Del Monte) | 1 cup | 140 |
| (Sun-Maid/Sunsweet) | 2-oz. serving | 150 |
| Frozen, sweetened | 1 cup | 325 |
| **APPLE BROWN BETTY** | 1 cup | 325 |

| Food and Description | Measure or Quantity | Calories |
|---|---|---|
| **APPLE BUTTER**: | | |
| (Bama) | 1 T. | 36 |
| (Home Brands) | 1 T. | 52 |
| (Smucker's) | 1 T. | 38 |
| (White House) | 1 T. | 38 |
| **APPLE CHERRY BERRY DRINK**, | | |
| canned (Lincoln) | 6 fl. oz. | 90 |
| **APPLE CIDER**: | | |
| Canned: | | |
| (Johanna Farms) | ½ cup | 56 |
| (Mott's) sweet | ½ cup | 59 |
| (Tree Top) | 6 fl. oz. | 90 |
| *Mix, *Country Time* | 8 fl. oz. | 98 |
| *APPLE CINNAMON SQUARES*, | | |
| cereal (Kellogg's) | ½ cup | 90 |
| **APPLE-CRANBERRY DRINK** | | |
| (Hi-C): | | |
| Canned | 6 fl. oz. | 90 |
| *Mix | 6 fl. oz. | 72 |
| **APPLE-CRANBERRY JUICE**, | | |
| canned (Lincoln) | 6 fl. oz. | 100 |
| **APPLE DRINK**: | | |
| Canned: | | |
| *Capri Sun,* natural | 6¾ fl. oz. | 90 |
| (Hi-C) | 6 fl. oz. | 92 |
| *Ssips* (Johanna Farms) | 8.45-fl.-oz. container | 130 |
| *Mix (Hi-C) | 6 fl. oz. | 72 |
| **APPLE DUMPLINGS**, frozen | | |
| (Pepperidge Farm) | 1 dumpling | 260 |
| **APPLE, ESCALLOPED**: | | |
| Canned (White House) | ½ cup (4.5 oz.) | 163 |
| Frozen (Stouffer's) | 4 oz. | 130 |
| **APPLE-GRAPE JUICE**, canned: | | |
| (Musselman's) | 6 fl. oz. | 82 |
| (Red Cheek) | 6 fl. oz. | 69 |
| *APPLE JACKS*, cereal (Kellogg's) | 1 cup (1 oz.) | 110 |
| **APPLE JAM** (Smucker's) | 1 T. | 53 |
| **APPLE JELLY**: | | |
| Sweetened: | | |
| (Bama) | 1 T. | 45 |
| (Home Brands) | 1 T. | 52 |
| (Smucker's) | 1 T. | 67 |
| Dietetic: | | |
| (Estee; Featherweight; | | |
| Louis Sherry) | 1 T. | 6 |
| (Diet Delight) | 1 T. | 12 |
| **APPLE JUICE**: | | |
| Canned: | | |
| (Borden) *Sippin' Pak* | 8.45-fl.-oz. container | 110 |

2

| Food and Description | Measure or Quantity | Calories |
|---|---|---|
| (Johanna Farms) *Tree Ripe* | 8.45-fl.-oz. container | 121 |
| (Lincoln) | 6 fl. oz. | 90 |
| (Red Cheek) | 6 fl. oz. | 85 |
| (Thank You Brand) | 6 fl. oz. | 82 |
| (Tree Top) regular | 6 fl. oz. | 90 |
| (White House) | 6 fl. oz. | 87 |
| Chilled (Minute Maid) | 6 fl. oz. | 91 |
| *Frozen: | | |
| (Minute Maid) | 6 fl. oz. | 91 |
| (Sunkist) | 6 fl. oz. | 59 |
| (Tree Top) | 6 fl. oz. | 90 |
| **APPLE JUICE DRINK,** canned | | |
| (Sunkist) | 8.5 fl. oz. | 140 |
| **APPLE PIE** (See PIE, Apple) | | |
| **APPLE RAISIN CRISP,** cereal | | |
| (Kellogg's) | ⅔ cup | 130 |
| **APPLE SAUCE:** | | |
| Regular: | | |
| (Del Monte) | ½ cup | 90 |
| (Hunt's) *Snack Pak:* | | |
| Regular | 4¼ oz. | 50 |
| Raspberry | 4¼ oz. | 80 |
| (Mott's): | | |
| Regular, jarred: | | |
| Regular | 6 oz. | 150 |
| Cinnamon | 6 oz. | 152 |
| Single-serve cups: | | |
| Regular | 4 oz. | 100 |
| Cherry | 3¾ oz. | 72 |
| Peach | 3¾ oz. | 75 |
| Strawberry | 3¾ oz. | 76 |
| (Thank You Brand) | ½ cup | 87 |
| (Tree Top) Natural | ½ cup | 60 |
| (White House) regular or chunky | ½ cup | 80 |
| Dietetic: | | |
| (Del Monte, Lite; Diet Delight) | ½ cup | 50 |
| (Mott's) Single-serve cups | 4 oz. | 53 |
| (S&W) *Nutradiet*, white or blue label | ½ cup | 55 |
| (Thank You Brand) | ½ cup | 54 |
| (White House) | ½ cup | 50 |
| **APPLE STRUDEL,** frozen | | |
| (Pepperidge Farm) | 3 oz. | 240 |
| **APRICOT:** | | |
| Fresh, whole | 1 apricot | 18 |
| Canned, regular pack: | | |
| (Del Monte) whole, or halves, peeled | ½ cup | 200 |
| (Stokely-Van Camp) | 1 cup | 220 |

3

| Food and Description | Measure or Quantity | Calories |
|---|---|---|
| Canned, dietetic, solids & liq.: | | |
| (Del Monte) Lite | ½ cup | 64 |
| (Diet Delight): | | |
| Juice pack | ½ cup | 60 |
| Water pack | ½ cup | 35 |
| (Featherweight): | | |
| Juice pack | ½ cup | 50 |
| Water pack | ½ cup | 35 |
| (Libby's) Lite | ½ cup | 60 |
| (S&W) *Nutradiet:* | | |
| Halves, white or blue label | ½ cup | 50 |
| Whole, juice | ½ cup | 40 |
| Dried: | | |
| (Del Monte; Sun-Maid; Sunsweet) | 2 oz. | 140 |
| **APRICOT & PINEAPPLE PRESERVE OR JAM:** | | |
| Sweetened: | | |
| (Home Brands) | 1 T. | 52 |
| (Smucker's) | 1 T. | 53 |
| Dietetic: | | |
| (Diet Delight; Louis Sherry) | 1 T. | 6 |
| (S&W) *Nutradiet* | 1 T. | 12 |
| **APRICOT LIQUEUR** (DeKuyper) | 1 fl. oz. | 82 |
| **APRICOT NECTAR:** | | |
| (Ardmore Farms) | 6 oz. | 94 |
| (Del Monte) | 6 fl. oz. | 100 |
| **APRICOT-PINEAPPLE NECTAR,** canned, dietetic (S&W) *Nutradiet,* blue label | 6 oz. | 35 |
| **APRICOT PRESERVE:** | | |
| Sweetened (Home Brands) | 1 T. | 51 |
| Dietetic (Estee) | 1 T. | 6 |
| ***ARBY'S:*** | | |
| Bac'n Cheddar Deluxe | 1 sandwich | 561 |
| Beef & Cheddar Sandwich | 1 sandwich | 490 |
| Chicken breast sandwich | 7¼-oz. sandwich | 592 |
| Croissant: | | |
| Bacon & egg | 1 croissant | 420 |
| Butter | 1 croissant | 220 |
| Chicken salad | 1 croissant | 460 |
| Ham & Swiss | 1 croissant | 330 |
| Mushroom & Swiss | 1 croissant | 340 |
| Sausage & egg | 1 croissant | 530 |
| French fries | 1½-oz. serving | 211 |
| Ham 'N Cheese | 1 sandwich | 353 |
| Potato cakes | 2 pieces | 201 |
| Potato, stuffed: | | |
| Broccoli & cheddar | 1 potato | 541 |
| Deluxe | 1 potato | 648 |

| Food and Description | Measure or Quantity | Calories |
|---|---|---|
| Mushroom & cheese | 1 potato | 506 |
| Taco | 1 potato | 619 |
| Roast Beef: | | |
| Regular | 5 oz. | 353 |
| Junior | 3 oz. | 218 |
| King | 6.7 oz. | 467 |
| Super | 9¼ oz. | 501 |
| Garden salad (no dressing) | 1 serving | 165 |
| Chef's salad (no dressing) | 1 serving | 235 |
| Cashew chicken salad (contains dressing) | 1 serving | 505 |
| Crackers | 1 packet | 25 |
| Croutons | 1 packet | 70 |
| Dressings: | | |
| Blue cheese | 1 packet | 390 |
| Buttermilk | 1 packet | 460 |
| Honey French | 1 packet | 350 |
| Light Italian | 1 packet | 25 |
| **ARTICHOKE:** | | |
| Boiled | 15-oz. artichoke | 187 |
| Canned (Cara Mia) marinated, drained | 6-oz. jar | 175 |
| Frozen (Birds Eye) deluxe | 3 oz. | 33 |
| **ASPARAGUS:** | | |
| Boiled | 1 spear (½" dia. at base) | 3 |
| Canned, regular pack, solid & liq.: | | |
| (Del Monte) spears, green or white | ½ cup | 20 |
| (Green Giant) | 8-oz. can | 46 |
| Canned, dietetic, solids & liq.: | | |
| (Diet Delight) | ½ cup | 16 |
| (Featherweight) cut spears | 1 cup | 40 |
| (S&W) *Nutradiet* | 1 cup | 40 |
| Frozen: | | |
| (Birds Eye): | | |
| Cuts | ⅓ pkg. | 22 |
| Spears | ⅓ pkg. | 23 |
| (Frosty Acres) | 3.3 oz. | 25 |
| (Green Giant) cuts, butter sauce | ½ cup | 70 |
| (McKenzie) | ⅓ pkg. | 25 |
| (Stouffer's) souffle | ⅓ pkg. | 115 |
| **ASPARAGUS PUREE,** canned (Larsen) | ½ cup | 22 |
| *AUNT JEMIMA SYRUP* (See SYRUP) | | |
| **AVOCADO** (Calavo) | ½ fruit, edible portion (3.05 oz.) | 155 |
| **AVOCADO PUREE** (Calavo) | ½ cup (8.1 oz.) | 411 |

5

| Food and Description | Measure or Quantity | Calories |
|---|---|---|
| *AWAKE* ( Birds Eye) | 6 fl. oz. | 84 |
| *AYDS:* | | |
| Butterscotch | 1 piece | 27 |
| Chocolate, chocolate mint, vanilla | 1 piece | 26 |

# B

| Food and Description | Measure or Quantity | Calories |
|---|---|---|
| **BACON,** broiled: | | |
| (Hormel) *Black Label* | 1 slice | 30 |
| (Oscar Mayer): | | |
| Regular slice | 6-gram slice | 35 |
| Center cut | 1 slice | 25 |
| Thick slice | 1 slice | 64 |
| **BACON BITS:** | | |
| *Bac\*Os* (Betty Crocker) | 1 tsp. | 13 |
| (French's) imitation | 1 tsp. | 6 |
| (Hormel) | 1 tsp. | 10 |
| (Libby's) crumbles | 1 tsp. | 8 |
| (Oscar Mayer) real | 1 tsp. | 6 |
| **BACON, CANADIAN,** unheated: | | |
| (Eckrich) | 1 oz. | 35 |
| (Hormel): | | |
| Regular | 1 slice | 45 |
| *Light & Lean* | 1 slice | 17 |
| (Oscar Mayer) 93% fat free: | | |
| Thin | .7-oz. slice | 30 |
| Thick | 1-oz. slice | 35 |
| **BACON, SIMULATED,** cooked: | | |
| (Oscar Mayer) *Lean'N Tasty*: | | |
| Beef | 1 strip | 48 |
| Pork | 1 strip | 54 |
| (Swift's) *Sizzlean*, pork | 1 strip | 35 |
| **BAGEL** (Lender's): | | |
| Plain: | | |
| Regular | 1 bagel | 150 |
| *Bagelette* | 1 bagel | 70 |
| Egg | 1 bagel | 150 |
| Onion | 1 bagel | 160 |
| Poppy seed | 1 bagel | 160 |
| Raisin & honey | 1 bagel | 200 |
| **BAKING POWDER:** | | |
| (Calumet) | 1 tsp. | 2 |
| (Davis) | 1 tsp. | 7 |
| (Featherweight) low sodium, cereal free | 1 tsp. | 8 |

| Food and Description | Measure or Quantity | Calories |
|---|---|---|
| **BAMBOO SHOOTS:** | | |
| Raw, trimmed | 4 oz. | 31 |
| Canned, drained (Chun King) | ½ cup | 32 |
| **BANANA,** medium (Dole) | 6.3-oz. banana (weighed unpeeled) | 101 |
| **BANANA EXTRACT** (Durkee) imitation | 1 tsp. | 15 |
| **BANANA NECTAR** (Libby's) | 6 fl. oz. | 60 |
| **BANANA PIE** (See PIE, Banana) | | |
| **BARBECUE SEASONING** (French's) | 1 tsp. | 6 |
| **BARBERA WINE** (Louis M. Martini) 12½% alcohol | 3 fl. oz. | 65 |
| **BARLEY,** pearled (Quaker Scotch) | ¼ cup | 172 |
| **BASIL** (French's) | 1 tsp. | 3 |
| **BASS:** | | |
| Baked, stuffed | 3½″ × 4½″ × 1½″ | 531 |
| Oven-fried | 8¾″ × 4½″ × ⅝″ | 392 |
| **BAY LEAF** (French's) | 1 tsp. | 5 |
| ***B & B LIQUEUR*** | 1 fl. oz. | 94 |
| **B.B.Q. SAUCE & BEEF,** frozen (Banquet) *Cookin' Bag,* sliced | 4-oz. serving | 100 |
| **BEAN, BAKED:** | | |
| (USDA): | | |
| With pork & molasses sauce | 1 cup | 382 |
| With pork & tomato sauce | 1 cup | 311 |
| Canned: | | |
| (Allens) *Wagon Master* | 1 cup | 260 |
| (B&M) *Brick Oven:* | | |
| Pea bean with pork in brown sugar sauce | 8 oz. | 300 |
| Red kidney bean in brown sugar sauce | 8 oz. | 290 |
| Vegetarian | 8 oz. | 250 |
| (Campbell): | | |
| Home style | 8-oz. can | 270 |
| With pork & tomato sauce | 8-oz. can | 240 |
| (Friend's): | | |
| Pea | 9-oz. serving | 360 |
| Yellow eye | 9-oz. serving | 360 |
| (Furman's) & pork, in tomato sauce | 8 oz. | 245 |
| (Grandma Brown's) | 8 oz. | 289 |
| (Hormel) *Short Orders,* with bacon | 7½-oz. can | 330 |
| (Hunt's) & pork | 8 oz. | 280 |
| **BEAN, BARBECUE** (Campbell) | 7⅞-oz. can | 678 |

| Food and Description | Measure or Quantity | Calories |
|---|---|---|
| **BEAN & BEEF BURRITO DINNER,** frozen (Swanson) | 15¼-oz. dinner | 720 |
| **BEAN, BLACK OR BROWN:** | | |
| Dry | 1 cup | 678 |
| Canned (Goya) black | 1 cup. | 250 |
| **BEAN, CHILI,** canned (Hunt's) | ½ cup | 90 |
| **BEAN, FAVA,** canned (Progresso) | 4 oz. | 90 |
| **BEAN & FRANKFURTER,** canned: | | |
| (Campbell) in tomato and molasses sauce | 7⅞-oz. can | 360 |
| (Hormel) *Short Orders,* 'n wieners | 7½-oz. can | 280 |
| **BEAN & FRANKFURTER DINNER,** frozen: | | |
| (Banquet) | 10-oz. dinner | 510 |
| (Swanson) | 12½-oz. dinner | 550 |
| **BEAN, GARBANZO,** canned: | | |
| Regular (Old El Paso) | ½ cup | 77 |
| Dietetic (S&W) *Nutradiet,* low sodium, green label | ½ cup | 105 |
| **BEAN, GREEN:** | | |
| Boiled, 1½" to 2" pieces, drained | ½ cup | 17 |
| Canned, regular pack, solids & liq.: | | |
| (Allen's): | | |
| Whole | ½ cup | 21 |
| With dry shelled beans | ½ cup | 40 |
| (Del Monte) | 4 oz. | 20 |
| (Green Giant) French or whole | ½ cup | 20 |
| (Larsen) *Freshlike* | ½ cup | 20 |
| Canned, dietetic, solids & liq.: | | |
| (Del Monte) No Salt Added | 4 oz. | 19 |
| (Diet Delight; S&W, *Nutradiet*) | ½ cup | 20 |
| (Larsen) *Fresh-Lite* | ½ cup | 20 |
| Frozen: | | |
| (Birds Eye): | | |
| Cut or French | ⅓ pkg. | 25 |
| French, with almonds | 3 oz. | 52 |
| Whole, deluxe | 3 oz. | 23 |
| (Frosty Acres) | 3 oz. | 30 |
| (Green Giant): | | |
| Cut or French, with butter sauce, regular | 3 oz. | 30 |
| Cut, *Harvest Fresh* | ⅓ of 8-oz. pkg. | 16 |
| (Larsen) | 3 oz. | 25 |
| (Seabrook Farms; Southland) | ⅓ pkg. | 29 |
| **BEAN, GREEN & MUSHROOM CASSEROLE** (Stouffer's) | ½ pkg. | 160 |
| **BEAN, GREEN, WITH POTATOES,** canned (Sunshine) solids & liq. | ½ cup | 34 |

| Food and Description | Measure or Quantity | Calories |
|---|---|---|
| **BEAN, ITALIAN:** | | |
| Canned (Del Monte) solids & liq. | 4 oz. | 25 |
| Frozen: | | |
| (Birds Eye) | 3 oz. | 31 |
| (Frosty Acres; Larsen) | 3 oz. | 30 |
| **BEAN, KIDNEY:** | | |
| Canned, regular pack, solids & liq.: | | |
| (Allen's) red | ½ cup | 110 |
| (Furman) red, fancy, light | ½ cup | 121 |
| (Goya): | | |
| Red | ½ cup | 115 |
| White | ½ cup | 100 |
| (Hunt's): | | |
| Regular | 4 oz. (3.5 oz.) | 120 |
| Small, red | ½ cup | 80 |
| (Progresso) | ½ cup | 95 |
| (Van Camp): | | |
| Light | 8 oz. | 194 |
| New Orleans style | 8 oz. | 188 |
| Red | 8 oz. | 213 |
| Canned, dietetic (S&W) *Nutradiet*, low sodium, | ½ cup | 90 |
| **BEAN, LIMA:** | | |
| Boiled, drained | ½ cup | 94 |
| Canned, regular pack, solids & liq.: | | |
| (Allen's): | | |
| Regular | ½ cup | 60 |
| Baby butter | ½ cup | 55 |
| (Del Monte) | 4 oz. | 70 |
| (Furman's) | ½ cup | 92 |
| (Larsen) *Freshlike* | ½ cup | 80 |
| (Sultana) butter bean | ¼ of 15-oz. can | 82 |
| Canned, dietetic (Featherweight) | ½ cup | 80 |
| Frozen: | | |
| (Birds Eye) baby | ⅓ pkg. | 126 |
| (Frosty Acres): | | |
| Baby | 3.3 oz. | 130 |
| Butter | 3.2 oz. | 140 |
| Fordhook | 3.3 oz. | 100 |
| (Green Giant): | | |
| In butter sauce | 3.3 oz | 83 |
| *Harvest Fresh* | 3 oz. | 60 |
| (Larsen) baby | 3.3 oz. | 130 |
| (Seabrook Farms): | | |
| Baby lima | ⅓ pkg. | 126 |
| Baby butter bean | ⅓ pkg. | 139 |
| Fordhooks | ⅓ pkg. | 98 |
| **BEAN, PINK,** canned | | |
| (Goya) | ½ cup | 115 |

10

| Food and Description | Measure or Quantity | Calories |
|---|---|---|
| **BEAN, PINTO:** | | |
| Canned, regular pack, solids & liq.: | | |
| (Gebhardt) | ⅓ of 15-oz. can | 245 |
| (Goya) | ½ cup (4 oz.) | 100 |
| Frozen (McKenzie) | 3.2-oz. serving | 160 |
| **BEAN, RED,** canned | | |
| (Goya) | ½ cup | 79 |
| **BEAN, REFRIED,** canned: | | |
| (Gebhardt) regular | 4 oz. | 130 |
| *Little Pancho,* & green chili | ½ cup | 80 |
| *Old El Paso:* | | |
| Plain | 4 oz. | 106 |
| With sausage | 4 oz. | 224 |
| (Rosarita): | | |
| Regular | 4 oz. | 130 |
| With green chilis | 4 oz. | 116 |
| **BEAN, ROMAN,** | | |
| canned (Goya) | ½ cup | 81 |
| **BEAN SALAD,** canned | | |
| (Green Giant) | ½ cup | 70 |
| **BEANS 'N FIXIN'S,** canned (Hunt's) | | |
| *Big John's:* | | |
| Beans | 3 oz. | 100 |
| Fixin's | 1 oz. | 50 |
| **BEAN SOUP** (See SOUP, Bean) | | |
| **BEAN SPROUT:** | | |
| Mung, raw | ½ lb. | 80 |
| Mung, boiled, drained | ¼ lb. | 32 |
| Soy, raw | ½ lb. | 104 |
| Soy, boiled, drained | ¼ lb. | 43 |
| Canned (drained) | ⅔ cup | 6 |
| **BEAN, WHITE,** canned | | |
| (Goya) solids & liq. | ½ cup | 105 |
| **BEAN, YELLOW OR WAX:** | | |
| Boiled, 1″ pieces, drained | ½ cup | 18 |
| Canned, regular pack, solids & liq.: | | |
| (Del Monte) cut or french | ½ cup | 18 |
| (Larsen) *Freshlike* | ½ cup | 25 |
| (Libby's) cut | 4 oz. | 23 |
| (Stokley-Van Camp) | ½ cup | 23 |
| Canned, dietetic (Featherweight) | | |
| cut, solids & liq. | ½ cup | 25 |
| Frozen (Frosty Acres) | 3 oz. | 25 |
| **BEAR CLAWS** (Dolly Madison) | | |
| cherry | 2¾-oz. piece | 270 |
| **BEEF,** choice grade, medium done: | | |
| Brisket, braised: | | |
| Lean & fat | 3 oz. | 350 |
| Lean only | 3 oz. | 189 |

| Food and Description | Measure or Quantity | Calories |
|---|---|---|
| Chuck, pot roast: | | |
| Lean & fat | 3 oz. | 278 |
| Lean only | 3 oz. | 182 |
| Fat, separable, cooked | 1 oz. | 207 |
| Filet mignon (See STEAK, sirloin, lean) | | |
| Flank, braised, 100% lean | 3 oz. | 167 |
| Ground: | | |
| Regular, raw | ½ cup | 303 |
| Regular, broiled | 3 oz. | 243 |
| Lean, broiled | 3 oz. | 186 |
| Rib: | | |
| Roasted, lean & fat | 3 oz. | 374 |
| Lean only | 3 oz. | 205 |
| Round: | | |
| Broiled, lean & fat | 3 oz. | 222 |
| Lean only | 3 oz. | 161 |
| Rump: | | |
| Broiled, lean & fat | 3 oz. | 295 |
| Lean only | 3 oz. | 177 |
| Steak, club, broiled: | | |
| One 8-oz. steak (weighed without bone before cooking) will give you: | | |
| Lean & fat | 5.9 oz. | 754 |
| Lean only | 3.4 oz. | 234 |
| Steak, porterhouse, broiled: | | |
| One 16-oz. steak (weighed with bone before cooking) will give you: | | |
| Lean & fat | 10.2 oz. | 1339 |
| Lean only | 5.9 oz. | 372 |
| Steak, ribeye, broiled: | | |
| One 10-oz. steak (weighed without bone before cooking) will give you: | | |
| Lean & fat | 7.3 oz. | 911 |
| Lean only | 3.8 oz. | 258 |
| Steak, sirloin, double-bone, broiled: | | |
| One 16-oz. steak (weighed with bone before cooking) will give you: | | |
| Lean & fat | 8.9 oz. | 1028 |
| Lean only | 5.9 oz. | 359 |
| One 12-oz. steak (weighed with bone before cooking) will give you: | | |
| Lean & fat | 6.6 oz. | 767 |
| Lean only | 4.4 oz. | 268 |

| Food and Description | Measure or Quantity | Calories |
|---|---|---|
| Steak, T-bone, broiled: | | |
| One 16-oz. steak (weighed with bone before cooking) will give you: | | |
| Lean & fat | 9.8 oz. | 1315 |
| Lean only | 5.5 oz. | 348 |
| **BEEF BOUILLON:** | | |
| (Herb-Ox): | | |
| Cube | 1 cube | 6 |
| Packet | 1 packet | 8 |
| *Lite-Line* (Borden) instant, low sodium | 1 tsp. | 12 |
| (MBT) | 1 packet | 14 |
| (Wyler's) | 1 cube | 6 |
| Low sodium (Featherweight) | 1 tsp. | 18 |
| **BEEF, CHIPPED:** | | |
| Cooked, home recipe | ½ cup | 188 |
| Frozen, creamed: | | |
| (Banquet) creamed: | 4-oz. pkg. | 100 |
| (Stouffer's) | 5½-oz. serving | 230 |
| **BEEF DINNER or ENTREE,** frozen: | | |
| (Armour): | | |
| *Classic Lites,* Steak Diane | 10-oz. meal | 270 |
| *Dinner Classics,* Sirloin tips | 11-oz. dinner | 290 |
| (Banquet): | | |
| American Favorites, chopped | 11-oz. dinner | 434 |
| Extra Helping, regular | 16-oz. dinner | 864 |
| (Blue Star) *Dining Light,* teriyaki | 8⅝-oz. dinner | 230 |
| (Conagra) *Light & Elegant,* Julienne | 8½-oz. entree | 260 |
| (La Choy) Fresh & Light, & broccoli with rice | 11-oz. meal | 260 |
| (Le Menu): | | |
| Chopped sirloin | 11½-oz. dinner | 390 |
| Yankee pot roast | 11-oz. dinner | 360 |
| (Morton) sliced | 10-oz. dinner | 215 |
| (Stouffer's): | | |
| *Lean Cuisine,* oriental with vegetables & rice | 8⅝-oz. meal | 250 |
| *Right Course:* | | |
| Dijon | 9½-oz. meal | 290 |
| Fiesta | 8⅞-oz. meal | 270 |
| (Swanson): | | |
| Regular, 4-compartment, chopped sirloin | 11½-oz. dinner | 350 |
| *Hungry Man:* | | |
| Chopped | 17¼-oz. dinner | 600 |
| Sliced | 12¼-oz. entree | 330 |

| Food and Description | Measure or Quantity | Calories |
|---|---|---|
| (Weight Watchers): | | |
| Beefsteak, 2-compartment meal | 8¹⁵⁄₁₆-oz. pkg. | 320 |
| Oriental | 10-oz. meal | 260 |
| **BEEF, DRIED,** canned: | | |
| (Hormel) | 1 oz. | 45 |
| (Swift) | 1 oz. | 47 |
| **BEEF GOULASH** (Hormel) | | |
| *Short Orders* | 7½-oz. can | 230 |
| **BEEF, GROUND, SEASONING MIX:** | | |
| *(Durkee): | | |
| Regular | 1 cup | 653 |
| With onion | 1 cup | 659 |
| (French's) with onion | 1⅛-oz. pkg. | 100 |
| **BEEF HASH, ROAST:** | | |
| Canned, *Mary Kitchen* (Hormel): | | |
| Regular | 7½-oz. serving | 350 |
| *Short Orders* | 7½-oz. can | 360 |
| Frozen (Stouffer's) | 10-oz. meal | 380 |
| **BEEF, PACKAGED** | | |
| (Carl Buddig) | 1 oz. | 38 |
| **BEEF, PEPPER ORIENTAL,** frozen | | |
| (La Choy) dinner | 12-oz. dinner | 250 |
| **BEEF PIE,** frozen: | | |
| (Banquet) | 8-oz. pie | 449 |
| (Morton) | 7-oz. pie | 430 |
| (Swanson): | | |
| Regular | 8-oz. pie | 400 |
| *Chunky* | 10-oz. pie | 530 |
| **BEEF PUFFS,** frozen (Durkee) | 1 piece | 47 |
| **BEEF ROLL** (Hormel) Lumberjack | 1 oz. | 101 |
| **BEEF, SHORT RIBS,** frozen: | | |
| (Armour) *Dinner Classics,* boneless | 10½-oz. dinner | 460 |
| (Stouffer's) boneless, with gravy | 9-oz. pkg. | 350 |
| **BEEF SOUP** (See SOUP, Beef) | | |
| **BEEF SPREAD, ROAST,** canned | | |
| (Underwood) | ½ of 4¾-oz. can | 140 |
| **BEEF STEAK, BREADED** (Hormel) frozen | 4-oz. serving | 370 |
| **BEEF STEW:** | | |
| Home recipe, made with lean beef chuck | 1 cup | 218 |
| Canned, regular pack: | | |
| *Dinty Moore* (Hormel): | | |
| Regular | 8-oz. serving | 210 |
| *Short Orders* | 7½-oz. can | 150 |
| (Libby's) | 7½-oz serving | 160 |

| Food and Description | Measure or Quantity | Calories |
|---|---|---|
| Canned, dietetic (Estee) | 7½-oz. serving | 210 |
| Frozen: | | |
| (Banquet) *Buffet Supper* | 2-lb. pkg. | 1016 |
| (Stouffer's) | 10-oz. serving | 305 |
| **BEEF STEW SEASONING MIX:** | | |
| *(Durkee) | 1 cup | 379 |
| (French's) | 1 pkg. | 150 |
| **BEEF STOCK BASE** (French's) | 1 tsp. | 8 |
| **BEEF STROGANOFF,** frozen: | | |
| (Armour) *Dinner Classics* | 10-oz. dinner | 320 |
| (Conagra) *Light & Elegant* | 9-oz. entree | 260 |
| (Le Menu) | 9¼ oz. dinner | 430 |
| (Stouffer's) with parsley noodles | 9¾ oz. | 390 |
| ***BEEF STROGANOFF SEASONING*** | | |
| **MIX** (Durkee) | 1 cup | 820 |
| **BEER & ALE:** | | |
| Regular: | | |
| *Black Horse Ale* | 8 fl. oz. | 108 |
| *Black Label* (Heilemann) | 8 fl. oz. | 68 |
| *Blatz* (Heilemann) | 8 fl. oz. | 93 |
| *Budweiser: Busch Bavarian* | 8 fl. oz. | 100 |
| *Michelob* | 8 fl. oz. | 113 |
| *Old Milwaukee* | 8 fl. oz. | 95 |
| *Pearl Premium* | 8 fl. oz. | 99 |
| *Schlitz* | 8 fl. oz. | 100 |
| *Stroh Bohemian* | 8 fl. oz. | 84 |
| Light or low carbohydrate: | | |
| *Budweiser Light; Natural light* | 8 fl. oz. | 75 |
| *Gablinger's* | 8 fl. oz. | 66 |
| *Michelob Light* | 8 fl. oz. | 90 |
| *Old Milwaukee* | 8 fl. oz. | 80 |
| *Pearl Light* | 8 fl. oz. | 60 |
| *Schlitz Light* | 8 fl. oz. | 64 |
| *Stroh Light* | 8 fl. oz. | 77 |
| **BEER, NEAR:** | | |
| *Goetz Pale* | 8 fl. oz. | 53 |
| (Metbrew) | 8 fl. oz. | 49 |
| **BEET:** | | |
| Boiled, whole | 2″-dia. beet | 16 |
| Boiled, sliced | ½ cup | 33 |
| Canned, regular pack, solids & liq.: | | |
| (Blue Boy) Harvard | ½ cup | 100 |
| (Del Monte) | | |
| Pickled | 4 oz. | 77 |
| Sliced | 4 oz. | 29 |
| (Greenwood) | | |
| Harvard | ½ cup | 70 |
| Pickled | ½ cup | 110 |

| Food and Description | Measure or Quantity | Calories |
|---|---|---|
| (Larsen) *Freshlike:* | | |
| Regular | ½ cup | 40 |
| Pickled | ½ cup | 100 |
| (Stokely-Van Camp) pickled | ½ cup | 95 |
| Canned, dietetic, solids & liq.: | | |
| (Blue Boy) whole | ½ cup | 39 |
| (Comstock) | ½ cup | 30 |
| (Featherweight) sliced | ½ cup | 45 |
| (Larsen) *Fresh-Lite* | ½ cup | 40 |
| (S&W) *Nutradiet,* sliced | ½ cup | 35 |
| **BEET PUREE,** canned (Larsen) | ½ cup | 45 |
| **BENEDICTINE LIQUEUR** (Julius Wile) | 1½ fl. oz. | 168 |
| **BERRY, MIXED, DRINK,** canned: | | |
| *Ssips* (Johanna Farms) | 8.45-fl.-oz. container | 130 |
| **BIG H,** burger sauce (Hellmann's) | 1 T. | 71 |
| **BIG MAC** (See *McDONALD'S*) | | |
| **BIG WHEEL** (Hostess) | 1 piece | 170 |
| **BISCUIT DOUGH** (Pillsbury): | | |
| Baking Powder, *1869 Brand* | 1 biscuit | 100 |
| Buttermilk: | | |
| Regular | 1 biscuit | 50 |
| *Ballard, Oven Ready* | 1 biscuit | 50 |
| Extra rich, *Hungry Jack* | 1 biscuit | 50 |
| Fluffy, *Hungry Jack* | 1 biscuit | 90 |
| *Butter Tastin', 1869 Brand* | 1 biscuit | 100 |
| Flaky, *Hungry Jack,* regular | 1 biscuit | 80 |
| *Oven Ready, Ballard* | 1 biscuit | 50 |
| **BITTERS** (Angostura) | 1 tsp. | 14 |
| **BLACKBERRY,** fresh, hulled | 1 cup | 84 |
| **BLACKBERRY JELLY:** | | |
| Sweetened (Home Brands) | 1 T. | 14 |
| Dietetic: | | |
| (Diet Delight) | 1 T. | 12 |
| (Featherweight) | 1 T. | 16 |
| **BLACKBERRY LIQUEUR** (Bols) | 1 fl. oz. | 95 |
| **BLACKBERRY PRESERVE OR JAM:** | | |
| Sweetened (Smucker's) | 1 T. | 53 |
| Dietetic: | | |
| (Estee; Louis Sherry) | 1 T. | 6 |
| (Featherweight) | 1 T. | 16 |
| (S&W) *Nutradiet* | 1 T. | 12 |
| **BLACKBERRY WINE** (Mogen David) | 3 fl. oz. | 135 |
| **BLACK-EYED PEAS:** | | |
| Canned: | | |
| (Allen's) | ½ cup | 100 |
| (Goya) | ½ cup | 105 |

| Food and Description | Measure or Quantity | Calories |
|---|---|---|
| (Trappey's) any style | ½ cup | 90 |
| Frozen: | | |
| (Birds Eye) | ⅓ pkg. | 133 |
| (Frosty Acres) | 3.3 oz. | 130 |
| (McKenzie; Seabrook Farms) | ⅓ pkg. | 130 |
| (Southland) | ⅓ of 16-oz. pkg. | 130 |
| **BLINTZ, frozen:** | | |
| (Empire Kosher): | | |
| Apple | 2½ oz. | 100 |
| Blueberry & cheese | 2½ oz. | 110 |
| Potato | 2½ oz. | 130 |
| (King Kold) cheese | 2½ oz. | 132 |
| **BLOODY MARY MIX:** | | |
| Dry (Bar-Tender's) | 1 serving | 26 |
| Liquid (Sacramento) | 5½-fl. oz. can | 39 |
| **BLUEBERRY, fresh, whole** | ½ cup | 45 |
| **BLUEBERRY PIE** (See PIE, Blueberry) | | |
| **BLUEBERRY PRESERVE OR JAM:** | | |
| Sweetened: | | |
| (Home Brands) | 1 T. | 52 |
| (Smucker's) | 1 T. | 53 |
| Dietetic (Louis Sherry) | 1 T. | 6 |
| ***BLUEBERRY SQUARES,*** cereal (Kellogg's) | ½ cup | 90 |
| **BLUEFISH,** broiled | 3½″ × 3″ × ½″ piece | 199 |
| ***BODY BUDDIES,*** cereal (General Mills): | | |
| Brown sugar & honey | 1 cup | 110 |
| Natural fruit flavor | ¾ cup | 110 |
| **BOLOGNA:** | | |
| (Eckrich): | | |
| Beef: | | |
| Regular, garlic | 1 oz. | 90 |
| Thick slice | 1½-oz. slice | 140 |
| German brand | 1-oz. slice | 80 |
| Meat, regular | 1-oz. slice | 90 |
| (Hebrew National) beef | 1 oz. | 90 |
| (Hormel): | | |
| Beef | 1-oz. slice | 85 |
| Meat | 1-oz. slice | 90 |
| (Ohse): | | |
| Regular | 1 oz. | 85 |
| 15% chicken | 1 oz. | 90 |
| (Oscar Mayer): | | |
| Beef | .5-oz. slice | 48 |
| Beef | 1-oz. slice | 90 |
| Beef Lebanon | .8-oz. slice | 47 |

17

| Food and Description | Measure or Quantity | Calories |
|---|---|---|
| Garlic beef | 1-oz. slice | 90 |
| Meat | 1-oz. slice | 90 |
| (Swift) *Light & Lean* | 1-oz. slice | 95 |
| **BOLOGNA & CHEESE:** | | |
| (Eckrich) | .7-oz. slice | 90 |
| (Oscar Mayer) | .8-oz. slice | 74 |
| **BONITO,** canned (Star-Kist): | | |
| Chunk | 6½-oz. can | 605 |
| Solid | 7-oz. can | 650 |
| ***BOO*BERRY,** cereal (General Mills) | 1 cup | 110 |
| **BORSCHT,** canned: | | |
| Regular: | | |
| (Gold's) | 8-oz. serving | 100 |
| (Manischewitz) | 8-oz. serving | 80 |
| (Mother's) old fashioned | 8-oz. serving | 90 |
| Dietetic or low calorie: | | |
| (Gold's) | 8-oz. serving | 20 |
| (Manischewitz) | 8-oz. serving | 20 |
| (Mother's): | | |
| Artificially sweetened | 8-oz. serving | 29 |
| Unsalted | 8-oz. serving | 107 |
| (Rokeach): | | |
| Diet | 8-oz. serving | 15 |
| Unsalted | 8-oz. serving | 103 |
| ***BOSCO*** (See SYRUP) | | |
| **BOYSENBERRY JELLY:** | | |
| Sweetened (Home Brands) | 1 T. | 15 |
| Dietetic (S&W) *Nutradiet,* red label | 1 T. | 12 |
| **BRAN:** | | |
| Crude | 1 oz. | 60 |
| Miller's (Elam's) | 1 oz. | 87 |
| **BRAN BREAKFAST CEREAL:** | | |
| (Kellogg's): | | |
| *All Bran* or *Bran Buds* | ⅓ cup | 70 |
| *Cracklin' Oat Bran* | ½ cup | 120 |
| 40% bran flakes | ¾ cup | 90 |
| Raisin | ¾ cup | 110 |
| (Loma Linda) | 1 oz. | 90 |
| (Nabisco) | ½ cup | 70 |
| (Post) 40% bran flakes | ⅔ cup | 107 |
| (Quaker) *Corn Bran* | ⅔ cup | 109 |
| (Ralston-Purina): | | |
| *Bran Chex* | ⅔ cup | 90 |
| Oat | 1 cup | 130 |
| **BRANDY** (See DISTILLED LIQUOR) | | |
| **BRANDY, FLAVORED** | | |
| (Mr. Boston): | | |
| Apricot | 1 fl. oz. | 94 |

| Food and Description | Measure or Quantity | Calories |
|---|---|---|
| Blackberry | 1 fl. oz. | 92 |
| Cherry | 1 fl. oz. | 87 |
| Ginger | 1 fl. oz. | 72 |
| Peach | 1 fl. oz. | 94 |
| **BRAUNSCHWEIGER:** | | |
| (Eckrich) chub | 1 oz. | 70 |
| (Oscar Mayer) chub | 1 oz. | 94 |
| (Swift) 8-oz. chub | 1 oz. | 109 |
| **BRAZIL NUT:** | | |
| Shelled | 4 nuts | 114 |
| Roasted (Fisher) salted | 1 oz. | 193 |
| **BREAD:** | | |
| Apple Cinnamon (Pritikin) | 1-oz. slice | 80 |
| Autumn Grain, *Merita* | 1-oz. slice | 75 |
| Barbecue, *Millbrook* | 1.23-oz. slice | 100 |
| Boston Brown | 3" × ¾" slice | 101 |
| *Bran'nola* (Arnold) | 1.3-oz. slice | 90 |
| Buttermilk: | | |
| *Butternut* | 1-oz. slice | 80 |
| *Holsum* | 1-oz. slice | 80 |
| *Sweetheart* | 1-oz. slice | 70 |
| Cinnamon (Pepperidge Farm) | .9-oz. slice | 85 |
| Cracked wheat: | | |
| (Pepperidge Farm) | .9-oz. slice | 70 |
| (Wonder) | 1-oz. slice | 75 |
| Crispbread, *Wasa:* | | |
| Rye, lite | .3-oz. slice | 30 |
| Sesame | .5-oz. slice | 50 |
| Date-nut roll (Dromedary) | 1-oz. slice | 80 |
| Egg, *Millbrook* | 1-oz. slice | 70 |
| Flatbread, *Ideal:* | | |
| Bran | .2-oz. slice | 19 |
| Extra thin | 1-oz. slice | 12 |
| Whole grain | .2-oz. slice | 19 |
| French: | | |
| *Eddy's,* regular or sour | 1-oz. slice | 70 |
| *Francisco* (Arnold) | 1-oz. slice | 70 |
| (Wonder) | 1-oz. slice | 71 |
| Garlic (Arnold) | 1-oz. slice | 80 |
| Hi-Fibre (Monk's) | 1-oz. slice | 50 |
| *Hillbilly, Holsum* | 1-oz. slice | 70 |
| *Hollywood,* dark | 1-oz. slice | 70 |
| Honey bran (Pepperidge Farm) | 1-oz. slice | 95 |
| Honey wheat berry (Arnold) | 1.1-oz. slice | 80 |
| Hunters Grain, *Country Farms* | 1.5-oz. slice | 120 |
| Italian (Arnold) *Francisco* | 1 slice | 70 |
| Low sodium, *Butternut* | 1-oz. slice | 80 |
| Multi-grain (Arnold) *Milk & Honey* | 1-oz. slice | 70 |
| Natural grains (Arnold) | .8-oz. slice | 60 |

**19**

| Food and Description | Measure or Quantity | Calories |
|---|---|---|
| Oat (Arnold) *Bran'nola* | 1.3-oz. slice | 110 |
| Oatmeal (Pepperidge Farm) | .9-oz. slice | 70 |
| Olympic Meal, *Holsum* | 1-oz. slice | 70 |
| Onion dill, Pritikin | 1-oz. slice | 70 |
| Pita (see *Sahara*, Thomas') | | |
| Protein (Thomas') | .7-oz. slice | 46 |
| Pumpernickel: | | |
| (Arnold) | 1-oz. slice | 80 |
| (Levy's) | 1.1-oz. slice | 80 |
| (Pepperidge Farm): | | |
| Regular | 1.1-oz. slice | 80 |
| Party | .2-oz. slice | 17 |
| Raisin: | | |
| (Arnold) tea | .9-oz. slice | 70 |
| (Monk's) & cinnamon | 1-oz. slice | 70 |
| (Pepperidge Farm) | 1 slice | 75 |
| Pritikin | 1-oz. slice | 70 |
| (Sun-Maid) | 1-oz. slice | 80 |
| *Roman Meal* | 1-oz. slice | 70 |
| Rye: | | |
| (Arnold) Jewish | 1.1-oz. slice | 80 |
| (Levy's) Real | 1.1-oz. slice | 80 |
| (Pepperidge Farm) family | 1.1-oz. slice | 85 |
| (Wonder) | 1-oz. slice | 70 |
| *Sahara* (Thomas') wheat or white | 1-oz. piece | 80 |
| Sourdough, *Di Carlo* | 1-oz. slice | 70 |
| Sunflower & bran (Monk's) | 1-oz. slice | 70 |
| Wheat (see also Cracked Wheat or Whole Wheat): | | |
| *America's Own*, cottage | 1-oz. slice | 70 |
| (Arnold): | | |
| *Bran'nola* | 1.3-oz. slice | 80 |
| *Less* or *Liteway* | .8-oz. slice | 40 |
| *Milk & Honey* | 1-oz. slice | 80 |
| *Fresh Horizons* | 1-oz. slice | 50 |
| *Fresh & Natural* | 1-oz. slice | 70 |
| *Home Pride* | 1-oz. slice | 70 |
| (Pepperidge Farm) sandwich | .8-oz. slice | 55 |
| (Wonder) family | 1-oz. slice | 70 |
| Wheatberry, *Home Pride*, honey | 1-oz. slice | 70 |
| White: | | |
| *America's Own*, cottage | 1-oz. slice | 70 |
| (Arnold): | | |
| *Brick Oven* | .8-oz. slice | 60 |
| Country | 1.3-oz. slice | 100 |
| *Less* | .8-oz. slice | 40 |
| *Milk & Honey* | 1-oz. slice | 80 |
| *Home Pride* | 1-oz. slice | 72 |
| (Monk's) | 1-oz. slice | 60 |

| Food and Description | Measure or Quantity | Calories |
|---|---|---|
| (Pepperidge Farm): | | |
| Regular | 1.2-oz. slice | 75 |
| Toasting | 1.2-oz. slice | 85 |
| (Wonder) regular | 1-oz. slice | 70 |
| Whole wheat: | | |
| (Arnold) *Stone Ground* | .8-oz. slice | 50 |
| (Monk's) | 1-oz. slice | 70 |
| (Pepperidge Farm) thin slice | 1 slice | 65 |
| (Wonder) 100% | 1-oz. slice | 69 |
| **BREAD, CANNED,** brown, plain or raisin (B&M) | ½" slice | 80 |
| **BREAD CRUMBS:** | | |
| (Contadina) seasoned | ½ cup | 211 |
| (Pepperidge Farm) | 1 oz. | 110 |
| ***BREAD DOUGH:** | | |
| Frozen: | | |
| (Pepperidge Farm): | | |
| Country rye or white | ⅒ loaf | 80 |
| Stone ground wheat | ⅒ loaf | 75 |
| (Rich's): | | |
| French | ⅟₂₀ loaf | 59 |
| Italian | ⅟₂₀ loaf | 60 |
| Refrigerated (Pillsbury): | | |
| French | 1" slice | 60 |
| Wheat or white | 1" slice | 80 |
| ***BREAD MIX:** | | |
| *Home Hearth*: | | |
| French | ⅜" slice | 85 |
| Rye or white | ⅜" slice | 75 |
| (Pillsbury): | | |
| Banana | ⅟₁₂ loaf | 170 |
| Cherry nut | ⅟₁₂ loaf | 180 |
| **BREAD PUDDING,** with raisins | ½ cup | 248 |
| **BREAD STICK** (Stella D'Oro): | | |
| Plain | 1 piece | 41 |
| Sesame | 1 piece | 50 |
| ***BREAD STICK DOUGH** (Pillsbury) | 1 piece | 100 |
| ***BREAKFAST DRINK** (Pillsbury) | 1 pouch | 290 |
| **BREAKFAST SQUARES** (General Mills) all flavors | 1 bar | 190 |
| **BROCCOLI:** | | |
| Boiled, with stalk | 1 stalk (6.3 oz.) | 47 |
| Boiled, ½" pieces | ½ cup | 20 |
| Frozen: | | |
| (Birds Eye): | | |
| In cheese sauce | 5 oz. | 132 |
| Chopped, cuts or florets | ⅓ pkg. | 26 |
| (Frosty Acres) | 3.3 oz. | 25 |
| (Green Giant): | | |
| Cuts, polybag | ½ cup (2 oz.) | 12 |

21

| Food and Description | Measure or Quantity | Calories |
|---|---|---|
| Spears in butter sauce, regular | 3⅓ oz. | 40 |
| Spears, mini, *Harvest Fresh* | ⅛ pkg. | 16 |
| (Larsen) | 3.3 oz. | 25 |
| (Seabrook Farms) chopped or spears | ⅓ pkg. | 30 |
| (Stouffer's) in cheese sauce | ½ of 9-oz. pkg. | 130 |
| **BROTH & SEASONING:** | | |
| (George Washington) | 1 packet | 5 |
| *Maggi* | 1 T. | 22 |
| **BRUNSWICK STEW,** canned | | |
| (Hormel) *Short Orders* | 7½-oz. can | 220 |
| **BRUSSELS SPROUT:** | | |
| Boiled | 3–4 sprouts | 28 |
| Frozen: | | |
| (Birds Eye): | | |
| Regular | ⅓ pkg. | 37 |
| Baby, with cheese sauce | 4½ oz. | 128 |
| (Frosty Acres) | 3.3 oz. | 35 |
| (Green Giant): | | |
| In butter sauce | 3.3 oz. | 40 |
| Polybag | ½ cup | 25 |
| **BUCKWHEAT,** cracked (Pocono) | 1 oz. | 104 |
| ***BUC*WHEATS,*** cereal (General Mills) | 1 oz. (¾ cup) | 110 |
| **BULGUR,** canned, seasoned | 4 oz. | 206 |
| ***BURGER KING:*** | | |
| Apple pie | 1 serving | 305 |
| Breakfast bagel sandwich: | | |
| Plain | 1 sandwich | 387 |
| Ham | 1 sandwich | 418 |
| Sausage | 1 sandwich | 621 |
| Breakfast Croissan'wich: | | |
| Bacon | 1 serving | 355 |
| Ham | 1 serving | 335 |
| Sausage | 1 serving | 538 |
| Cheeseburger: | | |
| Regular | 1 serving | 304 |
| Double: | | |
| Plain | 1 serving | 464 |
| bacon | 1 serving | 510 |
| Condiments: | | |
| Ketchup | 1 serving on sandwich | 11 |
| Mustard | 1 serving on sandwich | 2 |
| Pickles | 1 serving on sandwich | 0 |
| Chicken specialty sandwich: | | |
| Plain | 1 serving | 492 |

| Food and Description | Measure or Quantity | Calories |
|---|---|---|
| Condiments: | | |
| Lettuce | 1 serving on sandwich | 2 |
| Mayonnaise | 1 serving on sandwich | 194 |
| Chicken Tenders | 1 piece | 34 |
| Coffee, regular | 1 serving | 2 |
| Danish | 1 piece | 500 |
| Egg platter, scrambled: | | |
| Bacon | 1 serving | 68 |
| Croissant | 1 serving | 187 |
| Eggs | 1 serving | 119 |
| Hash browns | 1 serving | 162 |
| Sausage | 1 serving | 234 |
| French fries | 1 regular order | 227 |
| French toast sticks | 1 serving | 499 |
| Hamburger: | | |
| Plain | 1 burger | 262 |
| Condiments: | | |
| Ketchup | 1 serving on burger | 11 |
| Mustard | 1 serving on burger | 2 |
| Pickles | 1 serving on burger | 0 |
| Ham & cheese specialty: | | |
| Plain | 1 sandwich | 365 |
| Condiments: | | |
| Lettuce | 1 serving on sandwich | 3 |
| Mayonnaise | 1 serving on sandwich | 97 |
| Tomato | 1 serving on sandwich | 6 |
| Milk: | | |
| 2% low fat | 1 serving | 121 |
| Whole | 1 serving | 157 |
| Onion rings | 1 serving | 274 |
| Orange juice | 1 serving | 82 |
| Salad: | | |
| Chef | 1 salad | 180 |
| Chicken | 1 salad | 140 |
| Side | 1 salad | 20 |
| Salad dressing: | | |
| Regular: | | |
| Bleu cheese | 1 serving | 156 |
| House | 1 serving | 130 |
| 1000 Island | 1 serving | 117 |
| Dietetic, Italian | 1 serving | 14 |
| Shakes: | | |
| Chocolate | 1 shake | 374 |
| Vanilla | 1 shake | 334 |

| Food and Description | Measure or Quantity | Calories |
|---|---|---|
| Soft drink: | | |
| Sweetened: | | |
| *Pepsi-Cola* | 1 regular size | 159 |
| *7UP* | 1 regular size | 144 |
| Diet *Pepsi* | 1 regular size | 1 |
| *Whaler:* | | |
| Plain sandwich | 1 sandwich | 353 |
| Condiments: | | |
| Lettuce | 1 serving on sandwich | 1 |
| Tartar sauce | 1 serving on sandwich | 134 |
| *Whopper:* | | |
| Regular: | | |
| Plain | 1 sandwich | 452 |
| With cheese | 1 sandwich | 535 |
| Condiments: | | |
| Ketchup | 1 serving on sandwich | 17 |
| Lettuce | 1 serving on sandwich | 1 |
| Mayonnaise | 1 serving on sandwich | 146 |
| Onion | 1 serving on sandwich | 5 |
| Pickle | 1 serving on sandwich | 1 |
| Tomato | 1 serving on sandwich | 6 |
| Junior: | | |
| Plain | 1 sandwich | 262 |
| With cheese | 1 sandwich | 305 |
| Condiments: | | |
| Ketchup | 1 serving on sandwich | 8 |
| Lettuce | 1 serving on sandwich | 1 |
| Mayonnaise | 1 serving on sandwich | 48 |
| Pickle | 1 serving on sandwich | 0 |
| Tomato | 1 serving on sandwich | 3 |
| **BURGUNDY WINE:** | | |
| (Louis M. Martini) | 3 fl. oz. | 60 |
| (Paul Masson) | 3 fl. oz. | 70 |
| (Taylor) | 3 fl. oz. | 75 |
| **BURGUNDY WINE, SPARKLING:** | | |
| (Carlo Rossi) | 3 fl. oz. | 69 |

| Food and Description | Measure or Quantity | Calories |
|---|---|---|
| (B&G) | 3 fl. oz. | 69 |
| (Great Western) | 3 fl. oz. | 82 |
| (Taylor) | 3 fl. oz. | 78 |
| **BURRITO:** | | |
| *Canned (Del Monte) | 1 burrito | 310 |
| Frozen: | | |
| (Hormel): | | |
| Beef | 1 burrito | 220 |
| Cheese | 1 burrito | 250 |
| Hot chili | 1 burrito | 210 |
| (Fred's) *Little Juan:* | | |
| Bean & cheese | 5-oz. serving | 331 |
| Beef & potato | 5-oz. serving | 389 |
| Chili, red | 10-oz. serving | 799 |
| Red hot | 5-oz. serving | 433 |
| (Patio) | | |
| Dinner | 12-oz. dinner | 517 |
| Entree: | | |
| Regular | 5-oz. entree | 361 |
| Red chili | 5-oz. entree | 333 |
| (Swanson) bran & beef | 15¼-oz. meal | 720 |
| (Van de Kamp's) regular crispy fried | 6-oz. serving | 365 |
| **BURRITO FILLING MIX,** canned | | |
| (Del Monte) | ½ cup | 110 |
| **BURRITO SEASONING MIX** | | |
| (Lawry's) | 1 pkg. | 132 |
| **BUTTER:** | | |
| Regular: | | |
| (Breakstone) | 1 T. | 100 |
| (Meadow Gold) | 1 tsp. | 35 |
| Whipped (Breakstone) | 1 T. | 67 |
| **BUTTERSCOTCH MORSELS** | | |
| (Nestlé) | 1 oz. | 150 |
| **BUTTER SUBSTITUTE,** *Butter Buds:* | | |
| Dry or liquid | ⅛ oz. dry or 1 oz. liq. | 12 |
| Sprinkles | 1 tsp. | 140 |

# C

| Food and Description | Measure or Quantity | Calories |
|---|---|---|
| **CABBAGE:** | | |
| Boiled, until tender, without salt, drained | 1 cup | 29 |
| Canned, solids & liq.: | | |
| (Comstock) red | ½ cup | 60 |
| (Greenwood) | ½ cup | 60 |
| Frozen (Stouffer's) stuffed with meat, *Lean Cuisine* | 10¾-oz. meal | 220 |
| **CABERNET SAUVIGNON:** | | |
| (Louis M. Martini) | 3 fl. oz. | 62 |
| (Paul Masson) | 3 fl. oz. | 70 |
| ***CAFE COMFORT*, 55 proof** | 1 fl. oz. | 79 |
| **CAKE:** | | |
| Regular, non-frozen: | | |
| Plain, home recipe, with butter, with boiled white icing | ⅑ of 9″ square | 401 |
| Angel food: | | |
| Home recipe | ¹⁄₁₂ of 8″ cake | 108 |
| (Dolly Madison) | ⅙ of 10½-oz. cake | 120 |
| Apple (Dolly Madison) dutch, *Buttercrunch* | 1½-oz. piece | 170 |
| Butter streusel (Dolly Madison) *Buttercrumb* | 1½-oz. piece | 150 |
| Caramel, home recipe, with caramel icing | ⅑ of 9″ square | 322 |
| Carrot (Dolly Madison) *Lunch Cake* | 3¼-oz. serving | 350 |
| Chocolate, home recipe, with chocolate icing, 2-layer | ¹⁄₁₂ of 9″ cake | 365 |
| Chocolate (Dolly Madison) German, *Lunch Cake* | 3½-oz. piece | 440 |
| Cinnamon (Dolly Madison) *Buttercrumb* | 1½-oz. piece | 170 |
| Creme (Dolly Madison) *Lunch Cake* | ⅞-oz. cake | 90 |
| Cinnamon (Dolly Madison) Butter Crumb (Hostess) | 1¼-oz. cake | 130 |
| Fruit: | | |
| Home recipe, dark | ¹⁄₃₀ of 8″ loaf | 57 |

26

| Food and Description | Measure or Quantity | Calories |
|---|---|---|
| Home recipe, made with butter (Holland Honey Cake) | 1/30 of 8" loaf | 58 |
| unsalted | 1/14 of cake | 80 |
| Hawaiian Spice (Dolly Madison) *Lunch Cake* | 3½-oz. pkg. | 350 |
| Honey 'n spice (Dolly Madison) | 3¼-oz. serving | 330 |
| Pound, home recipe, traditional, made with butter | 3½" × 3½" slice | 123 |
| Raisin date loaf (Holland Honey Cake) low sodium | 1/14 of 13-oz. cake | 8 |
| Sponge, home recipe | 1/12 of 10" cake | 196 |
| White, home recipe, made with butter, without icing, 2-layer | 1/9 of 9" wide, 3" high cake | 353 |
| White (Dolly Madison) coconut layer | 1/12 of 30-oz. cake | 220 |
| Yellow, home recipe, made with butter, without icing, 2-layer | 1/19 of cake | 351 |
| Frozen: | | |
| Banana (Sara Lee) | 1/8 of 13¾-oz. cake | 175 |
| Butterscotch pecan (Pepperidge Farm) layer | 1/10 of 17-oz. cake | 160 |
| Carrot: | | |
| (Pepperidge Farm) | 1/8 of 11¼-oz. cake | 140 |
| (Weight Watchers) | 3-oz. serving | 180 |
| Cheesecake: | | |
| (Morton) *Great Little Desserts:* | | |
| Cherry | 6-oz. cake | 460 |
| Cream cheese | 6-oz. cake | 480 |
| Strawberry | 6-oz. cake | 470 |
| (Rich's) Viennese | 1/14 of 42-oz. cake | 230 |
| (Sara Lee): | | |
| Blueberry, *For 2* | ½ of 11.3-oz. cake | 425 |
| Cream cheese: | | |
| Regular | 1/3 of 10-oz. cake | 281 |
| Strawberry | 1/6 of 19-oz. cake | 223 |
| Strawberry, *For 2* | ½ of 11.3-oz. cake | 420 |
| (Weight Watchers): | | |
| Regular | 3.9-oz. serving | 200 |
| Strawberry | 3.9-oz. serving | 180 |
| Chocolate: | | |
| (Pepperidge Farm): | | |
| Layer, fudge | 1/10 of 17-oz. cake | 180 |
| Supreme, regular | ¼ of 11½-oz. cake | 310 |
| (Sara Lee): | | |
| Regular | 1/8 of 13¼-oz. cake | 199 |
| German | 1/8 of 12¼-oz. cake | 173 |
| (Weight Watchers) German | 2½ oz. | 200 |

| Food and Description | Measure or Quantity | Calories |
|---|---|---|
| Coconut (Pepperidge Farm) layer | ⅒ of 17-oz. cake | 180 |
| Coffee (Sara Lee): | | |
| Almond | ⅛ of 11¾-oz. cake | 165 |
| Apple | ⅛ of 15-oz. cake | 175 |
| Butter, *For 2* | ½ of 6½-oz. cake | 356 |
| Streusel, butter | ⅛ of 11½-oz. cake | 164 |
| Crumb (See ROLL OR BUN, Crumb) | | |
| Devil's food (Pepperidge Farm) layer | ⅒ of 17-oz. cake | 180 |
| Golden (Pepperidge Farm) layer | ⅒ of 17-oz. cake | 180 |
| *Grand Marnier* (Pepperidge Farm) | 1½ oz. | 160 |
| Lemon coconut (Pepperidge Farm) | ¼ of 12¼-oz. cake | 280 |
| Orange (Sara Lee) | ⅛ of 13¾-oz. cake | 179 |
| Pound: | | |
| (Pepperidge Farm) butter | ⅒ of 10¾-oz.cake | 130 |
| (Sara Lee): | | |
| Regular | ⅒ of 10¾-oz. cake | 125 |
| Banana nut | ⅒ of 11-oz. cake | 117 |
| Chocolate | ⅒ of 10¾-oz. cake | 122 |
| Spice (Weight Watchers) | 3-oz. serving | 170 |
| Strawberry cream (Pepperidge Farm) Supreme | ⅟₁₂ of 12-oz. cake | 190 |
| Strawberries'n cream, layer (Sara Lee) | ⅛ of 20½-oz. cake | 218 |
| Torte (Sara Lee): | | |
| Apples'n cream | ⅛ of 21-oz. cake | 203 |
| Fudge & nut | ⅛ of 15¾-oz. cake | 200 |
| Vanilla (Pepperidge Farm) layer | ⅒ of 17-oz. cake | 180 |
| Walnut, layer (Sara Lee) | ⅛ of 18-oz. cake | 210 |
| **CAKE OR COOKIE ICING** (Pillsbury): | | |
| All flavors except chocolate | 1 T. | 70 |
| Chocolate | 1 T. | 60 |
| **CAKE ICING:** | | |
| Butter pecan (Betty Crocker) *Creamy Deluxe* | ⅟₁₂ can | 160 |
| Caramel, home recipe | 4 oz. | 408 |
| Caramel pecan (Pillsbury) *Frosting Supreme* | ⅟₁₂ can | 160 |
| Cherry (Betty Crocker) *Creamy Deluxe* | ⅟₁₂ can | 160 |
| Chocolate: | | |
| (Betty Crocker) *Creamy Deluxe:* | | |
| Regular, chip or milk | ⅟₁₂ can | 170 |
| Sour cream | ⅟₁₂ can | 160 |

| Food and Description | Measure or Quantity | Calories |
|---|---|---|
| (Duncan Hines) regular or milk | ¹⁄₁₂ can | 163 |
| (Pillsbury) *Frosting Supreme,* fudge, nut or milk | ¹⁄₁₂ can | 150 |
| Coconut almond (Pillsbury) *Frosting Supreme* | ¹⁄₁₂ can | 150 |
| Cream cheese: | | |
| (Betty Crocker) *Creamy Deluxe* | ¹⁄₁₂ can | 170 |
| (Pillsbury) *Frosting Supreme* | ¹⁄₁₂ can | 160 |
| Double dutch (Pillsbury) *Frosting Supreme* | ¹⁄₁₂ can | 140 |
| Lemon (Pillsbury) *Frosting Supreme* | ¹⁄₁₂ can | 160 |
| Orange (Betty Crocker) *Creamy Deluxe* | ¹⁄₁₂ can | 160 |
| Rocky road minimorsels (Betty Crocker) *Creamy Deluxe* | ¹⁄₁₂ of can | 160 |
| Strawberry (Pillsbury) *Frosting Supreme* | ¹⁄₁₂ can | 160 |
| Vanilla: | | |
| (Betty Crocker) *Creamy Deluxe* | ¹⁄₁₂ can | 160 |
| (Duncan Hines) | ¹⁄₁₂ can | 163 |
| (Pillsbury) *Frosting Supreme,* regular or sour cream | ¹⁄₁₂ can | 160 |
| White: | | |
| Home recipe, boiled | 4 oz. | 358 |
| Home recipe, uncooked | 4 oz. | 426 |
| (Betty Crocker) *Creamy Deluxe* | ¹⁄₁₂ can | 160 |
| **\*CAKE ICING MIX:** | | |
| Regular: | | |
| Cherry (Betty Crocker) creamy | ¹⁄₁₂ pkg. | 170 |
| Chocolate: | | |
| Home recipe, fudge | ½ cup | 586 |
| (Betty Crocker) creamy: | | |
| Fluffy, almond fudge | ¹⁄₁₂ pkg. | 180 |
| Milk | ¹⁄₁₂ pkg. | 170 |
| (Pillsbury) *Frost It Hot* | ⅛ pkg. | 50 |
| Coconut almond (Pillsbury) | ¹⁄₁₂ pkg. | 160 |
| Coconut pecan: | | |
| (Betty Crocker) creamy | ¹⁄₁₂ pkg. | 160 |
| (Pillsbury) | ¹⁄₁₂ pkg. | 150 |
| Cream cheese & nuts (Betty Crocker) creamy | ¹⁄₁₂ pkg. | 160 |
| Lemon (Betty Crocker) creamy | ¹⁄₁₂ pkg. | 180 |
| Vanilla (Betty Crocker) creamy | ¹⁄₁₂ of pkg. | 190 |
| White: | | |
| (Betty Crocker) fluffy | ¹⁄₁₂ pkg. | 70 |
| (Betty Crocker) sour cream, creamy | ¹⁄₁₂ pkg. | 170 |

| Food and Description | Measure or Quantity | Calories |
|---|---|---|
| (Pillsbury) fluffy: | | |
| Regular | 1/12 pkg. | 60 |
| *Frost It Hot* | 1/8 pkg. | 50 |
| Dietetic (Pritikin) *Frostlite* | 1/12 pkg. | 25 |
| **CAKE MEAL** (Manischewitz) | 1/2 cup | 286 |
| **CAKE MIX:** | | |
| Regular: | | |
| *Apple (Pillsbury) *Streusel Swirl* | 1/16 of cake | 260 |
| Angel Food: | | |
| (Betty Crocker): | | |
| Chocolate or strawberry | 1/12 pkg. | 150 |
| Traditional | 1/12 pkg. | 130 |
| (Duncan Hines) | 1/12 pkg. | 124 |
| *Apple (Betty Crocker) *Cake Lovers Collection,* dutch | 1/12 of cake | 290 |
| Applesauce raisin (Betty Crocker) *Snackin' Cake* | 1/9 pkg. | 190 |
| *Banana (Pillsbury)*Pillsbury Plus* | 1/12 of cake | 250 |
| *Banana walnut (Betty Crocker) *Snackin' Cake* | 1/9 of cake | 200 |
| *Boston cream (Pillsbury) *Bundt* | 1/16 of cake | 270 |
| *Butter (Pillsbury) *Pillsbury Plus* | 1/12 of cake | 260 |
| *Butter Brickle (Betty Crocker) *Supermoist* | 1/12 of cake | 260 |
| *Butter pecan (Betty Crocker) *Supermoist* | 1/12 of cake | 250 |
| *Carrot (Betty Crocker): | | |
| *Cake Lovers Collection* | 1/12 of cake | 320 |
| *Supermoist* | 1/12 of cake | 260 |
| *Carrot'n spice (Pillsbury) *Pillsbury Plus* | 1/12 of cake | 260 |
| *Cheesecake: | | |
| (Jell-O) | 1/8 of 8" cake | 283 |
| (Royal) No Bake: | | |
| Lite | 1/8 of cake | 210 |
| Real | 1/8 of cake | 280 |
| *Cherry chip (Betty Crocker) *Supermoist* | 1/12 of cake | 180 |
| Chocolate: | | |
| (Betty Crocker): | | |
| *Cake Lovers Collection,* almond | 1/12 of cake | 360 |
| *Pudding | 1/6 of cake | 230 |
| *Snackin' Cake,* German | 1/9 of pkg. | 190 |
| *Stir 'N Frost:* | | |
| With chocolate frosting | 1/6 pkg. | 230 |

| Food and Description | Measure or Quantity | Calories |
|---|---|---|
| Fudge, with vanilla frosting | ⅙ pkg. | 230 |
| *Supermoist: | | |
| Butter recipe | 1/12 of cake | 270 |
| Chip | 1/12 of cake | 280 |
| Fudge | 1/12 of cake | 260 |
| Milk | 1/12 of cake | 260 |
| (Duncan Hines): | | |
| Deluxe | 1/12 of cake | 260 |
| Devil's food | 1/12 of cake | 280 |
| *(Pillsbury): | | |
| Bundt, tunnel of fudge | 1/16 of cake | 260 |
| Microwave: | | |
| Plain | ⅛ of cake | 210 |
| With chocolate frosting | ⅛ of cake | 300 |
| Pillsbury Plus: | | |
| Chocolate Chip | 1/12 of cake | 270 |
| Dark | 1/12 of cake | 250 |
| German | 1/12 of cake | 250 |
| *Cinnamon (Pillsbury) | | |
| Streusel Swirl: | | |
| Regular | 1/16 of cake | 260 |
| Microwave | ⅛ of cake | 240 |
| Coffee cake: | | |
| *(Aunt Jemima) | ⅛ of cake | 170 |
| *(Pillsbury) Apple cinnamon | ⅛ of cake | 240 |
| Devil's food: | | |
| *(Betty Crocker) Supermoist | 1/12 of cake | 270 |
| (Duncan Hines) deluxe | 1/12 pkg. | 190 |
| *(Pillsbury) Pillsbury Plus | 1/12 of cake | 270 |
| Fudge (See Chocolate) | | |
| Golden chocolate chip | | |
| (Betty Crocker) Snackin' Cake | ⅑ pkg. | 190 |
| Lemon: | | |
| (Betty Crocker) Supermoist | 1/12 cake | 260 |
| *(Pillsbury): | | |
| Bundt, tunnel of | 1/16 cake | 270 |
| Streusel Swirl | 1/16 cake | 270 |
| *Lemon blueberry (Pillsbury) | | |
| Bundt | 1/16 cake | 200 |
| *Marble (Betty Crocker) | | |
| Supermoist | 1/12 cake | 260 |
| *Pineapple creme (Pillsbury) | | |
| Bundt | 1/16 cake | 260 |
| Pound: | | |
| *(Betty Crocker) golden | 1/12 cake | 200 |
| *(Dromedary) | ½" slice | 150 |
| Spice (Betty Crocker), | | |
| Supermoist | 1/12 cake | 250 |

| Food and Description | Measure or Quantity | Calories |
|---|---|---|
| Strawberry, *(Pillsbury) *Pillsbury Plus* | 1/12 cake | 260 |
| *Upside down (Betty Crocker) pineapple | 1/9 cake | 250 |
| *Vanilla (Betty Crocker) golden, *Supermoist* | 1/12 of cake | 280 |
| White: | | |
| *(Betty Crocker): | | |
|   *Stir 'N Frost,* with chocolate frosting | 1/6 cake | 220 |
|   *Supermoist* | 1/12 cake | 250 |
| (Duncan Hines) deluxe | 1/12 pkg. | 188 |
| Yellow: | | |
| *(Betty Crocker) *Supermoist* | 1/12 cake | 250 |
| (Duncan Hines) deluxe | 1/12 pkg. | 188 |
| *(Pillsbury): | | |
|   *Microwave, plain | 1/8 of cake | 220 |
|   *Pillsbury Plus* | 1/12 of cake | 260 |
| *Dietetic: | | |
| (Estee) any flavor | 1/10 of cake | 100 |
| (Pritikin) *Batterlite,* unfrosted | 1/10 of cake | 90 |
| **CAMPARI,** 45 proof | 1 fl. oz. | 66 |
| **CANDY, REGULAR:** | | |
| Almond, Jordan (Banner) | 1¼-oz. box | 154 |
| *Almond Joy* (Peter Paul Cadbury) | 1.5-oz. bar | 220 |
| Apricot Delight (Sahadi) | 1 oz. | 100 |
| *Baby Ruth* | 2-oz. piece | 260 |
| *Bar None* (Hershey's) | 1½ oz. | 240 |
| *Bonkers!* any flavor | 1 piece | 20 |
| *Breath Savers* (Life Savers) | 1 piece | 8 |
| *Butterfinger* | 2-oz. bar | 260 |
| *Butternut* (Hollywood Brands) | 2¼-oz. bar | 310 |
| Caramel: | | |
|   *Caramel Flipper* (Wayne) | 1 oz. | 128 |
|   *Caramel Nip* (Pearson) | 1 piece | 30 |
| *Charleston Chew* | 2-oz. piece | 240 |
| Cherry, chocolate-covered (*Welch's*) dark | 1 piece | 90 |
| Chocolate bar: | | |
|   Brazil nut (Cadbury's) | 2 oz. | 310 |
|   Caramello (Cadbury's) | 2 oz. | 280 |
|   *Crunch* (Nestlé) | 1 1/16-oz. bar | 160 |
|   Hazelnut (Cadbury's) | 2 oz. | 310 |
|   Milk: | | |
|     (Cadbury's) | 2 oz. | 300 |
|     (Hershey's) | 1.65-oz. bar | 250 |
|     (Nestlé) | .35-oz. bar | 53 |
|     (Nestlé) | 1 1/16-oz. bar | 159 |

| Food and Description | Measure or Quantity | Calories |
|---|---|---|
| *Special Dark* (Hershey's) | 1.45-oz. bar | 220 |
| Chocolate bar with almonds: | | |
| (Cadbury's) | 2 oz. | 310 |
| (Hershey's) milk | 1.55-oz. bar | 250 |
| (Nestlé) | 1 oz. | 160 |
| *Chocolate Parfait* (Pearson) | 1 piece | 30 |
| Chocolate, Petite (Andes) | 1 piece | 26 |
| *Chuckles* | 1 oz. | 92 |
| *Clark Bar* | 1.5-oz. bar | 201 |
| *Coffee Nip* (Pearson) | 1 piece | 30 |
| *Coffioca Parfait* (Pearson) | 1 piece | 30 |
| Creme de Menthe (Andes) | 1 piece | 25 |
| *Crispy Bar* (Clark) | 1¼-oz. bar | 187 |
| *Crows* (Mason) | 1 piece | 11 |
| *Dutch Treat Bar* (Clark) | 1¹/₁₆-oz. bar | 160 |
| Eggs (Peter Paul Cadbury) creme | 1 oz. | 136 |
| *5th Avenue* (Hershey's) | 1.93-oz. bar | 270 |
| Fruit bears (Flavor Tree) assorted | ½ of 2.1-oz. envelope | 117 |
| Fruit circus (Flavor Tree) | ½ of 2.1-oz. envelope | 117 |
| Fruit roll (Flavor Tree): | | |
| Apple or cherry | ¾-oz. roll | 75 |
| Strawberry | ¾-oz. roll | 74 |
| Fudge (Nabisco) bar | 1 piece | 85 |
| *Good Stuff* (Nab) | 1.8-oz. piece | 250 |
| Halvah (Sahadi) original and marble | 1 oz. | 150 |
| Hard (Jolly Rancher): | | |
| All flavors except butterscotch | 1 piece | 23 |
| Butterscotch | 1 piece | 25 |
| *Hollywood* | 1½-oz. bar | 185 |
| Jelly bean, *Chuckles* | .5 oz. | 55 |
| Jelly rings, *Chuckles* | 1 piece | 37 |
| Jujubes, *Chuckles* | .5 oz. | 55 |
| *Ju Jus:* | | |
| Assorted | 1 piece | 7 |
| Coins or raspberries | 1 piece | 15 |
| *Kisses* (Hershey's) | 1 piece | 24 |
| *Kit Kat* | 1.6-oz. bar | 250 |
| *Krackel Bar* | .35-oz. bar | 52 |
| *Krackel Bar* | 1.6-oz. bar | 250 |
| Licorice: | | |
| (Switzer) bars, bites or stix: | | |
| Black | 1 oz. | 94 |
| Cherry or strawberry | 1 oz. | 98 |
| Chocolate | 1 oz. | 97 |
| Twist: | | |
| Black (American Licorice Co.) | 1 piece | 27 |
| Black (Curtiss) | 1 piece | 27 |

| Food and Description | Measure or Quantity | Calories |
|---|---|---|
| Red (American Licorice Co.) | 1 piece | 33 |
| *Life Savers* | 1 piece | 10 |
| Lollipops (Life Savers) | 1 pop | 45 |
| *Mallo Cup* (Boyer) | 9/16-oz. piece | 54 |
| Malted milk balls (Brach's) | 1 piece | 9 |
| *Mars Bar* (M&M/Mars) | 1.7-oz. bar | 240 |
| Marshmallow (Campfire) | 1 oz. | 111 |
| *Mary Jane* (Miller): | | |
| Small size | 1.4 oz. | 19 |
| Large size | 1½-oz. bar | 110 |
| *Milk Duds* (Clark) | ¾-oz. box | 89 |
| *Milk Shake* (Hollywood Brands) | 2.4-oz. bar | 300 |
| *Milky Way* (M&M/Mars) | 2.24-oz. bar | 290 |
| Mint or peppermint: | | |
| After dinner (Richardson): | | |
| Jelly center | 1 oz. | 104 |
| Regular | 1 oz. | 109 |
| Chocolate covered (Richardson) | 1 oz. | 106 |
| *Junior* mint pattie (Nabisco) | 1 piece | 10 |
| *Mint Parfait* (Andes) | 1 piece | 27 |
| Peppermint Pattie (Nabisco) | 1 piece | 55 |
| *York,* pattie (Peter Paul Cadbury) | 1¼-oz. serving | 160 |
| *M & M's:* | | |
| Peanut | 1.83-oz. pkg. | 270 |
| Plain | 1.69-oz. pkg. | 240 |
| *Mounds* (Peter Paul Cadbury) | 1.65-oz. serving | 230 |
| *Mr. Goodbar* (Hershey's) | 1.8-oz. bar | 300 |
| *Munch Bar* (M&M/Mars) | 1.42-oz. bar | 220 |
| *My Buddy* (Tom's) | 1.8-oz. piece | 250 |
| Naturally Nut & Fruit Bar (Planters) almond/apricot | 1 oz. | 140 |
| *$100,000 Bar* (Nestlé) | 1¼-oz. bar | 175 |
| Orange slices, *Chuckles* | 1 oz. | 110 |
| *Park Avenue* (Tom's) | 1.8-oz. bar | 230 |
| *Payday* (Hollywood Brands) regular | 1.9-oz. bar | 250 |
| Peanut bar (Planters) | 1.6 oz. | 240 |
| Peanut, chocolate-covered: | | |
| (Curtiss) | 1 piece | 5 |
| (Nabisco) | 1 piece | 11 |
| Peanut butter cup: | | |
| (Boyer) | 1.5-oz. pkg. | 148 |
| (Reese's) | .9-oz. cup | 140 |
| *Peanut Butter Pals* (Tom's) | 1.3-oz. serving | 200 |
| Peanut crunch bar (Sahadi) | ¾-oz. bar | 110 |
| Peanut Parfait (Andes) | 1 piece | 28 |
| *Peanut Plank* (Tom's) | 1.7-oz. piece | 230 |
| *Peanut Roll* (Tom's) | 1.75-oz. piece | 230 |

| Food and Description | Measure or Quantity | Calories |
|---|---|---|
| *Powerhouse* (Peter Paul Cadbury) | 2 oz. | 260 |
| Raisin, chocolate-covered: | | |
| (Nabisco) | 1 piece | 5 |
| *Raisinets* (BB) | 1 oz. | 140 |
| *Reese's Pieces* (Hershey's) | 1.95-oz. pkg. | 270 |
| *Reggie Bar* | 2-oz. bar | 290 |
| *Rolo* (Hershey's) | 1 piece | 30 |
| *Royals,* mint chocolate | | |
| (M&M/Mars) | 1.52-oz. pkg. | 212 |
| Sesame Crunch (Sahadi) | ¾-oz. bar | 110 |
| *Skor* (Hershey's) | 1.4-oz. bar | 220 |
| *Snickers* | 2-oz. bar | 290 |
| Spearmint leaves, *Chuckles* | 1 oz. | 110 |
| *Starburst* (M&M/Mars) | 1-oz. serving | 120 |
| *Sugar Babies* (Nabisco) | 1.6-oz. pkg. | 180 |
| *Sugar Daddy* (Nabisco) | | |
| caramel sucker | 1.4-oz. pop | 150 |
| *Sugar Mama* (Nabisco) | ¾-oz. pop | 90 |
| *Summit* bar (M&M/Mars) | 1 bar | 115 |
| Taffy: | | |
| Salt water (Brach's) | 1 piece | 31 |
| Turkish (Bonomo) | 1 oz. | 108 |
| *3 Musketeers* | .8-oz. bar | 99 |
| *3 Musketeers* | 2.1-oz. bar | 260 |
| *Ting-A-Ling* (Andes) | 1 piece | 24 |
| *Tootsie Roll:* | | |
| Chocolate | .23-oz. midgee | 26 |
| Chocolate | 1/16-oz. bar | 72 |
| Chocolate | 1-oz. bar | 115 |
| Flavored | .6-oz. square | 19 |
| Pop, all flavors | .49-oz. pop | 55 |
| Pop drop, all flavors | 4.7-gram piece | 19 |
| *Twix* Cookie bar (M&M/Mars) | 1¾-oz. serving | 246 |
| Peanut butter cookie bar | | |
| (M&M/Mars) | 1¾-oz. serving | 261 |
| *Twizzlers* | 1 oz. | 100 |
| *Whatchamacallit* (Hershey's) | 1.8-oz. bar | 260 |
| *Wispa* (Peter Paul Cadbury) | 1 oz. | 150 |
| *World Series Bar* | 1 oz. | 128 |
| *Y & S Bites* | 1 oz. | 100 |
| *Zagnut Bar* (Clark) | .7-oz. bar | 85 |
| *Zero* (Hollywood Brands) | 2-oz. bar | 210 |
| **CANDY, DIETETIC:** | | |
| Carob bar, *Joan's Natural:* | | |
| Coconut | 3-oz. bar | 516 |
| Fruit & nut | 3-oz. bar | 559 |
| Honey bran | 3-oz. bar | 487 |
| Peanut | 3-oz. bar | 521 |

| Food and Description | Measure or Quantity | Calories |
|---|---|---|
| Chocolate or chocolate-flavored bar: | | |
| (Estee): | | |
| Coconut, fruit & nut or milk | .2-oz. square | 30 |
| Crunch | .2-oz. square | 22 |
| (Louis Sherry) coffee or orange flavored | .2-oz. square | 22 |
| *Estee-ets*, with peanuts (Estee) | 1 piece | 7 |
| Gum drops (Estee) any flavor | 1 piece | 6 |
| *Gummy Bears* (Estee) | 1 piece | 5 |
| Hard candy: | | |
| (Estee) assorted fruit | 1 piece | 12 |
| (Louis Sherry) | 1 piece | 12 |
| Mint: | | |
| (Estee) | 1 piece | 4 |
| (Sunkist): | | |
| Mini mint | 1 piece | 1 |
| Roll mint | 1 piece | 4 |
| Peanut brittle (Estee) | ¼ oz. | 35 |
| Peanut butter cup (Estee) | 1 cup | 40 |
| Raisins, chocolate-covered (Estee) | 1 piece | 5 |
| **CANNELLONI,** frozen: | | |
| (Blue Star) *Dining Light*, cheese | 9-oz. dinner | 261 |
| (Celentano) | 12-oz. pkg. | 380 |
| (Stouffer's) beef & pork with mornay sauce, *Lean Cuisine* | 9⅝-oz. pkg. | 260 |
| (Weight Watchers) one-compartment | 13-oz. meal | 450 |
| **CANTALOUPE,** cubed | ½ cup (3 oz.) | 24 |
| **CAPERS** (Crosse & Blackwell) | 1 tsp. | 2 |
| *CAP'N CRUNCH,* cereal (Quaker): | | |
| Regular | ¾ cup | 121 |
| Crunchberry | ¾ cup | 120 |
| Peanut butter | ¾ cup | 127 |
| **CAPOCOLLO** (Hormel) | 1 oz. | 80 |
| **CARAWAY SEED** (French's) | 1 tsp. | 8 |
| *CARL'S JR. RESTAURANT:* | | |
| Bacon | 2 strips (10 grams) | 50 |
| Cake, chocolate | 3.2-oz. piece | 380 |
| *California Roast Beef 'n Swiss Sandwich* | 7.2-oz. sandwich | 360 |
| Cheese: | | |
| American | .6-oz. slice | 63 |
| Swiss | .6-oz. slice | 57 |
| Chicken sandwich: | | |
| *Charbroiler BBQ* | 6.3-oz. sandwich | 320 |
| *Charbroiler Club* | 8.2-oz. sandwich | 510 |
| Cookie, chocolate chip | 2¼-oz. piece | 330 |

| Food and Description | Measure or Quantity | Calories |
|---|---|---|
| Danish | 3.5-oz. piece | 300 |
| Eggs, scrambled | 2.4-oz. serving | 120 |
| Fish sandwich, filet | 7.9-oz. sandwich | 550 |
| French toast dips, excluding syrup | 4.7-oz. serving | 480 |
| Hamburger: | | |
| Plain: | | |
| *Famous Star* | 8.1-oz. serving | 590 |
| *Happy Star* | 3.0-oz. serving | 220 |
| *Old Time Star* | 5.9-oz. serving | 400 |
| *Super Star* | 10.6-oz. serving | 770 |
| *Cheeseburger, Western Bacon:* | | |
| Regular | 7½-oz. serving | 630 |
| Double | 10.4-oz. serving | 890 |
| Hot cake, with margarine, excluding syrup | 5.5-oz. serving | 360 |
| Milk, 2% lowfat | 10 fl. oz. | 175 |
| Muffins: | | |
| Blueberry | 3.5-oz. piece | 256 |
| Bran | 4-oz. piece | 220 |
| English, with margarine | 2-oz. piece | 180 |
| Onion rings | 3.2-oz. order | 310 |
| Orange juice, small | 8 fl. oz. | 94 |
| Potato: | | |
| Baked: | | |
| Bacon & cheese | 14.1-oz. serving | 650 |
| Broccoli & cheese | 14-oz. serving | 470 |
| Cheese | 14.2-oz. serving | 550 |
| Fiesta | 15.2-oz. serving | 550 |
| Lite | 9.8-oz. serving | 250 |
| Sour cream & chive | 10.4-oz. serving | 350 |
| French fries | Regular order (6 oz.) | 360 |
| Hash brown nuggets | 3-oz. serving | 170 |
| Salad dressing: | | |
| Regular: | | |
| Blue cheese | 2-oz. serving | 150 |
| House | 2-oz. serving | 186 |
| 1000 Island | 2-oz. serving | 231 |
| Dietetic, Italian | 2-oz. serving | 80 |
| Sausage patty | 1.5-oz. piece | 190 |
| Shake | 1 regular size | 353 |
| Soft drink: | | |
| Sweetened | 1 regular size | 243 |
| Dietetic | 1 regular size | 2 |
| Soup: | | |
| Broccoli, cream of | 1 serving | 140 |
| Chicken & noodle | 1 serving | 80 |
| Clam chowder, Boston | 1 serving | 140 |
| Vegetable, mixed | 1 serving | 70 |

| Food and Description | Measure or Quantity | Calories |
|---|---|---|
| Steak Sandwich, *Country Fried Sunrise Sandwich:* | 7.2-oz. serving | 610 |
| Bacon | 4.5-oz. serving | 370 |
| Sausage | 6.1-oz. serving | 500 |
| Tea, iced | 1 regular drink | 2 |
| Zucchini | 4.3-oz. serving | 300 |
| **CARNATION DO-IT-YOURSELF DIET PLAN** | 2 scoops | 110 |
| **CARNATION INSTANT BREAKFAST:** | | |
| Bar: | | |
| Chocolate chip | 1 bar | 200 |
| Peanut butter crunch | 1 bar | 180 |
| Packets, all flavors | 1 packet | 130 |
| **CARROT:** | | |
| Raw | 5½″ × 1″ piece | 21 |
| Boiled, slices | ½ cup | 24 |
| Canned, regular pack, solids & liq.: | | |
| (Del Monte) sliced or whole | ½ cup | 30 |
| (Larsen) *Freshlike* | ½ cup | 30 |
| (Libby's) | ½ cup | 20 |
| Canned, dietetic pack, solids & liq., (S&W) *Nutradiet,* green label | ½ cup | 30 |
| Frozen: | | |
| (Birds Eye) deluxe | 2.7 oz. | 32 |
| (Frosty Acres) | 3.3 oz. | 40 |
| (Green Giant) cuts, in butter sauce | ½ cup | 80 |
| (Larsen) | 3.3 oz. | 40 |
| (Seabrook Farms) | ⅓ pkg. | 39 |
| **CASABA MELON** | 1-lb. melon | 61 |
| **CASHEW NUT:** | | |
| (Eagle Snacks) honey roast | 1 oz. | 170 |
| (Fisher): | | |
| Dry roasted | 1 oz. | 156 |
| Honey, salted | 1 oz. | 150 |
| Oil roasted | 1 oz. | 159 |
| (Planters): | | |
| Dry roasted | 1 oz. | 160 |
| Honey roasted | 1 oz. | 170 |
| Oil roasted | 1 oz. | 170 |
| **CATFISH,** frozen (Mrs. Paul's) breaded & fried, fingers | 4 oz. | 250 |
| **CATSUP:** | | |
| Regular: | | |
| (Del Monte) | 1 T. | 17 |
| (Heinz) | 1 T. | 18 |
| (Hunt's) | 1 T. | 16 |
| (Smucker's) | 1 T. | 21 |

| Food and Description | Measure or Quantity | Calories |
|---|---|---|
| Dietetic or low calorie: | | |
| (Del Monte) No Salt Added | 1 T. | 15 |
| (Featherweight) | 1 T. | 6 |
| (Heinz) lite | 1 T. | 18 |
| (Hunt's) | 1 T. | 20 |
| **CAULIFLOWER:** | | |
| Raw or boiled buds | ½ cup | 14 |
| Frozen: | | |
| (Birds Eye) regular | 3.3 oz. | 23 |
| (Frosty Acres) | 3.3 oz. | 25 |
| (Green Giant) in cheese sauce | ⅓ of 10-oz. pkg. | 50 |
| (Larsen) | 3.3 oz. | 25 |
| **CAVATELLI**, frozen | | |
| (Celentano) | ⅓ of 16-oz. pkg. | 270 |
| **CAVIAR:** | | |
| Pressed | 1 oz. | 90 |
| Whole eggs | 1 T. | 42 |
| **CELERY:** | | |
| 1 large outer stalk | 8″ × 1½″ at root end | 7 |
| Diced or cut | ½ cup | 9 |
| Frozen (Larsen) | 3½ oz. | 14 |
| Salt (French's) | 1 tsp. | 12 |
| Seed (French's) | 1 tsp. | 11 |
| *CERTS* | 1 piece | 6 |
| **CERVELAT** (Hormel) Viking | 1-oz. serving | 90 |
| **CHABLIS WINE:** | | |
| (Almaden) light | 3 fl. oz. | 42 |
| (Carlo Rossi) | 3 fl. oz. | 66 |
| (Gallo) white or pink | 3 fl. oz. | 60 |
| (Louis M. Martini) | 3 fl. oz. | 59 |
| (Paul Masson): | | |
| Regular | 3 fl. oz. | 71 |
| Light | 3 fl. oz. | 45 |
| **CHAMPAGNE:** | | |
| (Bollinger) | 3 fl. oz. | 72 |
| (Great Western): | | |
| Regular | 3 fl. oz. | 71 |
| Brut | 3 fl. oz. | 74 |
| Pink | 3 fl. oz. | 81 |
| (Taylor) dry | 3 fl. oz. | 78 |
| **CHARDONNAY WINE** | | |
| (Louis M. Martini) | 3 fl. oz. | 63 |
| **CHARLOTTE RUSSE,** | | |
| homemade recipe | 4 oz. | 324 |
| *CHEERIOS,* cereal, regular or | | |
| honey & nut | 1 oz. | 110 |
| **CHEESE:** | | |
| American or cheddar: | | |
| Cube, natural | 1″ cube | 68 |

| Food and Description | Measure or Quantity | Calories |
|---|---|---|
| (Borden) | 1 oz. | 110 |
| (Churny) lite, cheddar, mild | 1 oz. | 80 |
| (Dorman's) *Chedda-De Lite* | 1 oz. | 90 |
| (Kraft): | | |
| American Singles | 1 oz. | 90 |
| Cheddar | 1 oz. | 110 |
| Old English | 1 oz. | 110 |
| *Laughing Cow,* natural | 1 oz. | 110 |
| (Polly-O) cheddar, shredded | 1 oz. | 110 |
| (Sargento): | | |
| Midget, regular or sharp | 1 oz. | 114 |
| Shredded, non-dairy | 1 oz. | 90 |
| *Wispride* | 1 oz. | 115 |
| Blue: | | |
| (Frigo) | 1 oz. | 100 |
| (Kraft) | 1 oz. | 100 |
| (Sargento) cold pack or crumbled | 1 oz. | 100 |
| Bonbino, *Laughing Cow,* natural | 1 oz. | 103 |
| Brick (Sargento) | 1 oz. | 105 |
| Brie (Sargento) *Danish Danko* | 1 oz. | 80 |
| Burgercheese (Sargento) *Danish Danko* | 1 oz. | 106 |
| Camembert (Sargento) *Danish Danko* | 1 oz. | 88 |
| Colby: | | |
| (Churny) lite | 1 oz. | 80 |
| (Featherweight) low sodium | 1 oz. | 100 |
| (Kraft) | 1 oz. | 110 |
| (Pauly) low sodium | 1 oz. | 115 |
| (Sargento) shredded or sliced | 1 oz. | 112 |
| Cottage: | | |
| Unflavored: | | |
| (Bison): | | |
| Regular | 1 oz. | 29 |
| Dietetic | 1 oz. | 22 |
| (Borden): | | |
| Regular, 4% milkfat | ½ cup | 120 |
| *Lite-Line,* 1.5% milkfat | ½ cup | 90 |
| (Breakstone's) smooth & creamy | 1 oz. | 27 |
| (Dairylea) | 1 oz. | 30 |
| (Friendship) | 1 oz. | 30 |
| (Johanna): | | |
| Large or small curd | ½ cup | 120 |
| No salt added | ½ cup | 90 |
| (Light n' Lively) | 1 oz. | 20 |
| (Sealtest) | 1 oz. | 30 |
| Flavored (Friendship) | | |
| Dutch apple | 1 oz. | 31 |

| Food and Description | Measure or Quantity | Calories |
|---|---|---|
| Cream, plain, unwhipped: | | |
| (Frigo) | 1 oz. | 100 |
| (Kraft) *Philadelphia Brand*: | | |
| Regular | 1 oz. | 100 |
| Light | 1 oz. | 60 |
| Edam: | | |
| (Churny) *May-Bud* | 1 oz. | 100 |
| (House of Gold) | 1 oz. | 100 |
| (Kaukauna) | 1 oz. | 100 |
| (Kraft) | 1 oz. | 90 |
| *Laughing Cow* | 1 oz. | 100 |
| Farmers: | | |
| (Churny) *May-Bud* | 1 oz. | 90 |
| *Dutch Garden Brand* | 1 oz. | 100 |
| (Kaukauna) | 1 oz. | 100 |
| (Sargento) | 1 oz. | 72 |
| *Wispride* | 1 oz. | 100 |
| Feta (Sargento) cups | 1 oz. | 76 |
| Gjetost (Sargento) Norwegian | 1 oz. | 118 |
| Gouda: | | |
| (Churny) *May-Bud*, lite | 1 oz. | 81 |
| (Kaukauna) | 1 oz. | 100 |
| *Laughing Cow* | 1 oz. | 110 |
| (Sargento) baby, caraway or smoked | 1 oz. | 101 |
| *Wispride* | 1 oz. | 100 |
| Grated (Polly-O) | 1 oz. | 130 |
| Gruyère, *Swiss Knight* | 1 oz. | 100 |
| Havarti (Sargento): | | |
| Creamy | 1 oz. | 90 |
| Creamy, 60% mild | 1 oz. | 117 |
| Hoop (Friendship) natural | 1 oz. | 21 |
| Hot pepper (Sargento) | 1 oz. | 112 |
| Jarlsberg (Sargento) Norwegian | 1 oz. | 100 |
| Kettle Moraine (Sargento) | 1 oz. | 100 |
| Limburger (Sargento) natural | 1 oz. | 100 |
| Monterey Jack: | | |
| (Churny) lite | 1 oz. | 80 |
| (Frigo) | 1 oz. | 100 |
| (Kaukauna) | 1 oz. | 110 |
| (Sargento) midget, Longhorn, shredded or sliced | 1 oz. | 106 |
| Mozzarella: | | |
| (Fisher) part skim milk | 1 oz. | 90 |
| (Kraft) | 1 oz. | 80 |
| (Polly-O): | | |
| Fior di Latte | 1 oz. | 80 |
| Part skim milk | 1 oz. | 80 |
| Smoked | 1 oz. | 85 |

| Food and Description | Measure or Quantity | Calories |
|---|---|---|
| Whole milk: | | |
|     Regular or shredded | 1 oz. | 90 |
|     Old fashioned, regular | 1 oz. | 70 |
| (Sargento): | | |
|     Bar, rounds, shredded regular | | |
|     or with spices, sliced for | | |
|     pizzas or square | 1 oz. | 79 |
|     Whole milk | 1 oz. | 100 |
| Muenster: | | |
|     (Dorman's) | 1 oz. | 110 |
|     (Kaukauna) | 1 oz. | 110 |
|     (Sargento) red rind | 1 oz. | 104 |
|     *Wispride* | 1 oz. | 100 |
| Nibblin Curds (Sargento) | 1 oz. | 114 |
| Parmesan: | | |
|     (Frigo): | | |
|       Grated | 1 T. | 23 |
|       Whole | 1 oz. | 110 |
|     (Polly-O) grated | 1 oz. | 130 |
|     (Sargento): | | |
|       Grated | 1 T. | 27 |
|       Wedge | 1 oz. | 110 |
| Pizza (Sargento) shredded or sliced | 1 oz. | 90 |
| Pot (Sargento) regular, | | |
|     French onion or garlic | 1 oz. | 30 |
| Provolone: | | |
|     (Frigo) | 1 oz. | 90 |
|     *Laughing Cow:* | | |
|       Cube | ⅙ oz. | 12 |
|       Wedge | ¾ oz. | 55 |
|     (Sargento) sliced | 1 oz. | 100 |
| Ricotta: | | |
|     (Frigo) part skim milk | 1 oz. | 43 |
|     (Polly-O): | | |
|       Lite | 1 oz. | 40 |
|       Part skim milk | 1 oz. | 45 |
|       Whole milk | 1 oz. | 50 |
|     (Sargento): | | |
|       Part skim milk | 1 oz. | 39 |
|       Whole milk | 1 oz. | 49 |
| Romano: | | |
|     (Polly-O) grated | 1 oz. | 130 |
|     (Sargento) wedge | 1 oz. | 110 |
| Roquefort, natural | 1 oz. | 104 |
| Samsoe (Sargento) Danish | 1 oz. | 79 |
| Scamorze (Frigo) | 1 oz. | 79 |
| Semisoft, *Laughing Cow:* | | |
|     *Babybel* | 1 oz. | 90 |
|     *Bonbel* | 1 oz. | 100 |

| Food and Description | Measure or Quantity | Calories |
|---|---|---|
| Slim Jack (Dorman's) | 1 oz. | 90 |
| Stirred curd (Frigo) | 1 oz. | 110 |
| String (Sargento) | 1 oz. | 90 |
| Swiss: | | |
| (Churny) lite | 1 oz. | 90 |
| (Dorman's) | 1 oz. | 100 |
| (Fisher) natural | 1 oz. | 100 |
| (Frigo) domestic | 1 oz. | 100 |
| (Sargento) domestic or Finland, sliced | 1 oz. | 107 |
| Taco (Sargento) shredded | 1 oz. | 105 |
| Washed curd (Frigo) | 1 oz. | 110 |
| **CHEESE FONDUE,** *Swiss Knight* | 1 oz. | 110 |
| **CHEESE FOOD:** | | |
| American or cheddar: | | |
| (Borden) *Lite Line* | 1 oz. | 50 |
| (Fisher) *Ched-O-Mate* or *Sandwich-Mate* | 1 oz. | 90 |
| (Weight Watchers) colored or white | 1-oz. slice | 50 |
| *Wispride:* | | |
| Regular | 1 oz. | 100 |
| & port wine | 1 oz. | 100 |
| *Cheez-ola* (Fisher) | 1 oz. | 90 |
| *Chef's Delight* (Fisher) | 1 oz. | 70 |
| *Count Down* (Pauly) | 1 oz. | 40 |
| Cracker snack (Sargento) | 1 oz. | 90 |
| Garlic & herbs, *Wispride* | 1 oz. | 90 |
| Jalapeño (Borden) *Lite Line* | 1 oz. | 50 |
| Loaf, *Count Down* (Pauly) | 1 oz. | 100 |
| Low sodium (Borden) *Lite Line* | 1 oz. | 70 |
| Monterey Jack (Borden) *Lite Line* | 1 oz. | 50 |
| *Mun-chee* (Pauly) | 1 oz. | 100 |
| Pimiento (Pauly) | .8-oz. slice | 73 |
| Pizza-Mate (Fisher) | 1 oz. | 90 |
| Swiss: | | |
| (Borden) *Lite Line* | 1 oz. | 50 |
| (Kraft) reduced fat | 1 oz. | 90 |
| **CHEESE PUFFS,** frozen (Durkee) | 1 piece | 59 |
| **CHEESE SPREAD:** | | |
| American or cheddar: | | |
| (Fisher) | 1 oz. | 80 |
| *Laughing Cow* | 1 oz. | 72 |
| (Nabisco) *Easy Cheese* | 1 tsp. | 16 |
| Blue, *Laughing Cow* | 1 oz. | 72 |
| Cheese'n Bacon (Nabisco) *Easy Cheese* | 1 tsp. | 16 |
| Gruyère, *Laughing Cow, La Vache Que Rit,* reduced calorie | 1 oz. | 46 |

| Food and Description | Measure or Quantity | Calories |
|---|---|---|
| Provolone, *Laughing Cow* | 1 oz. | 72 |
| Sharp (Pauly) | .8 oz. | 77 |
| Swiss, process (Pauly) | .8 oz. | 76 |
| *Velveeta* (Kraft) | 1 oz. | 80 |
| **CHEESE STRAW,** frozen (Durkee) | 1 piece | 29 |
| **CHENIN BLANC WINE** | | |
| (Louis M. Martini) | 3 fl. oz. | 62 |
| **CHERRY,** sweet: | | |
| Fresh, with stems | ½ cup | 41 |
| Canned, regular pack (Del Monte) | | |
| dark, solids & liq. | ½ cup | 50 |
| Canned, dietetic, solids & liq.: | | |
| (Diet Delight) with pits, | | |
| water pack | ½ cup | 70 |
| (Featherweight) dark, water pack | ½ cup | 60 |
| (Thank You Brand) | ½ cup | 61 |
| **CHERRY, CANDIED** | 1 oz. | 96 |
| **CHERRY DRINK:** | | |
| Canned: | | |
| (Hi-C) | 6 fl. oz. | 100 |
| (Lincoln) cherry berry | 6 fl. oz. | 100 |
| *Ssips* (Johanna Farms) | 8.45-fl.-oz. container | 130 |
| *Mix (Hi-C) | 6 fl. oz. | 72 |
| ***CHERRY HEERING*** | | |
| (Hiram Walker) | 1 fl. oz. | 80 |
| **CHERRY JELLY:** | | |
| Sweetened (Smucker's) | 1 T. | 53 |
| Dietetic: | | |
| (Dia-Mel) | 1 T. | 6 |
| (Featherweight) | 1 T. | 16 |
| **CHERRY LIQUEUR** (DeKuyper) | 1 fl. oz. | 75 |
| **CHERRY PRESERVES OR JAM:** | | |
| Sweetened (Smucker's) | 1 T. | 53 |
| Dietetic (Estee) | 1 T. | 6 |
| **CHESTNUT,** fresh, in shell | ¼ lb. | 220 |
| **CHEWING GUM:** | | |
| Sweetened: | | |
| *Bazooka,* bubble | 1 slice | 18 |
| *Beechies* | 1 piece | 6 |
| *Beech Nut; Beeman's Big Red; Black Jack; Clove; Doublemint; Freedent; Juicy Fruit; Spearmint* (Wrigley's); *Teaberry* | 1 stick | 10 |
| *Bubble Yum* | 1 piece | 25 |
| *Dentyne* | 1 piece | 4 |
| *Extra* (Wrigley's) | 1 piece | 8 |
| *Fruit Stripe,* regular | 1 piece | 9 |
| *Hubba Bubba* (Wrigley's) | 1 piece | 23 |

| Food and Description | Measure or Quantity | Calories |
|---|---|---|
| Dietetic: | | |
| *Bubble Yum* | 1 piece | 20 |
| *Care Free,* regular | 1 piece | 8 |
| (Clark; *Care\*Free*) | 1 piece | 7 |
| (Estee) bubble or regular | 1 piece | 5 |
| *Extra* (Wrigley's) cinnamon or spearmint | 1 piece | 8 |
| (Featherweight) bubble or regular | 1 piece | 4 |
| **CHEX,** cereal (Ralston Purina): | | |
| Corn | 1 cup | 110 |
| Rice | 1 cup | 110 |
| Wheat | ⅔ cup | 100 |
| Wheat & raisins | ¾ cup | 130 |
| **CHIANTI WINE:** | | |
| (Italian Swiss Colony) | 3 fl. oz. | 83 |
| (Louis M. Martini) | 3 fl. oz. | 90 |
| **CHICKEN:** | | |
| Broiler, cooked, meat only | 3 oz. | 116 |
| Fryer, fried, meat & skin | 3 oz. | 212 |
| Fryer, fried, meat only | 3 oz. | 178 |
| Fryer, fried, 2½-lb. chicken (weighed with bone before cooking) will give you: | | |
| Back | 1 back | 139 |
| Breast | ½ breast | 160 |
| Leg or drumstick | 1 leg | 87 |
| Neck | 1 neck | 127 |
| Rib | 1 rib | 41 |
| Thigh | 1 thigh | 122 |
| Wing | 1 wing | 82 |
| Fried skin | 1 oz. | 119 |
| Hen & cock: | | |
| Stewed, dark meat only | 3 oz. | 176 |
| Stewed, diced | ½ cup | 139 |
| Stewed, light meat only | 3 oz. | 153 |
| Stewed, meat & skin | 3 oz. | 269 |
| Roaster, roasted, dark or light meat, without skin | 3 oz. | 156 |
| **CHICKEN À LA KING:** | | |
| Home recipe | 1 cup | 468 |
| Canned (Swanson) | ½ of 10½-oz. can | 180 |
| Frozen: | | |
| (Banquet) *Cookin' Bag* | 4-oz. pkg. | 110 |
| (Blue Star) *Dining Lite,* with rice | 9½-oz. entree | 290 |
| (Le Menu) | 10¼-oz. dinner | 320 |
| (Stouffer's) with rice | 9½-oz. pkg. | 290 |
| (Weight Watchers) | 9-oz. pkg. | 230 |

| Food and Description | Measure or Quantity | Calories |
|---|---|---|
| **CHICKEN, BONED,** canned: | | |
| Regular: | | |
| (Hormel) chunk, breast | 6¾-oz. serving | 350 |
| (Swanson) chunk: | | |
| Mixin' chicken | 2½ oz. | 130 |
| White | 2½ oz. | 90 |
| Low sodium (Featherweight) | 2½ oz. | 154 |
| **CHICKEN BOUILLON:** | | |
| (Herb-Ox): | | |
| Cube | 1 cube | 6 |
| Packet | 1 packet | 12 |
| (Wyler's) | 1 cube | 8 |
| Low sodium: | | |
| (Featherweight) | 1 tsp. | 18 |
| *Lite-Line* (Borden) | 1 tsp. | 12 |
| **CHICKEN, CREAMED,** frozen (Stouffer's) | 6½ oz. | 300 |
| **CHICKEN DINNER OR ENTREE:** | | |
| Canned: | | |
| (Hunt's) *Minute Gourmet Microwave Entree Maker:* | | |
| Barbecued: | | |
| Without chicken | 3.1 oz. | 150 |
| *With chicken | 6.8 oz. | 320 |
| Sweet & sour: | | |
| Without chicken | 4.1 oz. | 130 |
| *With chicken | 7.8 oz. | 300 |
| (Swanson) & dumplings | 7½ oz. | 220 |
| Frozen: | | |
| (Armour): | | |
| *Classics Lite:* | | |
| Burgundy | 10½-oz.dinner | 210 |
| Sweet & sour | 10½-oz. dinner | 240 |
| *Dinner Classics:* | | |
| Fricassee | 11¾-oz. dinner | 340 |
| Milan | 11½-oz. dinner | 320 |
| (Banquet): | | |
| American Favorites | 11-oz. dinner | 359 |
| Family Entrees | 32-oz. pkg. | 1720 |
| (Blue Star) *Dining Lite,* glazed | 8½-oz. dinner | 243 |
| (Celentano): | | |
| Parmigiana | 9-oz. meal | 310 |
| Primavera | 11½-oz. pkg. | 270 |
| (Chun King) & walnuts, crunchy | 13-oz. meal | 117 |
| (Conagra) *Light & Elegant:* | | |
| Cheese | 8¾-oz. entree | 293 |
| Parmigiana | 8-oz. entree | 260 |

46

| Food and Description | Measure or Quantity | Calories |
|---|---|---|
| (Green Giant): | | |
| Baked: | | |
| In BBQ sauce with corn on the cob | 1 meal | 350 |
| Stir fry and garden vegetables | 10-oz. entree | 250 |
| (La Choy) Fresh and Lite: | | |
| Almond with rice and vegetables | 9¾-oz. meal | 270 |
| Oriental, spicy | 9¾-oz. meal | 270 |
| (Le Menu) sweet & sour | 11¼-oz. dinner | 450 |
| (Morton): | | |
| Regular: | | |
| Boneless | 11-oz. dinner | 329 |
| Fried | 11-oz. pkg. | 431 |
| Light, boneless | 11-oz. dinner | 250 |
| (Stouffer's): | | |
| Regular: | | |
| Cashew in sauce, with rice | 9½-oz. meal | 380 |
| Divan | 8½-oz. meal | 320 |
| *Lean Cuisine:* | | |
| Glazed with vegetable rice | 8½-oz. serving | 270 |
| & vegetables with vermicelli | 12¾-oz. serving | 260 |
| *Right Course:* | | |
| Italiano, with fettucini & vegetables | 9⅝-oz. meal | 280 |
| Sesame | 10-oz. meal | 320 |
| Tenderloin, in barbecue sauce with rice pilaf | 8¾-oz. meal | 270 |
| (Swanson): | | |
| Regular: | | |
| & dumplings | 7½-oz. meal | 220 |
| Fried, 4-compartment: | | |
| Barbecue flavor | 9¼-oz. dinner | 560 |
| Dark meat | 10¼-oz. dinner | 610 |
| *Hungry Man:* | | |
| Boneless | 17½-oz. dinner | 670 |
| Parmigiana | 20-oz. dinner | 810 |
| (Tyson): | | |
| A l'orange | 8¼-oz. meal | 300 |
| Français | 8¾-oz. meal | 350 |
| Parmigiana | 11¾-oz. meal | 450 |
| (Weight Watchers): | | |
| Cacciatore | 10-oz. serving | 290 |
| Imperial | 9¼-oz. meal | 240 |
| Parmigiana | 8-oz. serving | 290 |
| **CHICKEN, FRIED,** frozen: | | |
| (Banquet) assorted | 2-lb. pkg. | 1625 |
| (County Pride) southern fried, patties | 3 oz. | 232 |

47

| Food and Description | Measure or Quantity | Calories |
|---|---|---|
| (Swanson) *Plump & Juicy:* | | |
| Assorted | 3¼-oz. serving | 270 |
| Breast portions | 4½-oz. serving | 350 |
| Nibbles | 3¼-oz. serving | 300 |
| Take-out style | 3¼-oz. serving | 270 |
| *CHICKEN HELPER* (General Mills): | | |
| & dumplings | ⅕ of pkg. | 530 |
| & mushrooms | ⅕ of pkg. | 470 |
| Teriyaki | ⅕ of pkg. | 480 |
| CHICKEN & NOODLES, frozen: | | |
| (Green Giant) twin pouch, with vegetables | 9-oz. pkg. | 365 |
| (Stouffer's): | | |
| Escalloped | 5¾-oz. serving | 252 |
| Paprikash | 10½-oz. serving | 391 |
| CHICKEN NUGGETS, frozen | | |
| (Banquet) regular | 12-oz. pkg. | 932 |
| CHICKEN, PACKAGED: | | |
| (Carl Buddig) smoked | 1 oz. | 50 |
| (Louis Rich) breast, oven roasted | 1-oz. slice | 40 |
| CHICKEN PATTY, frozen (Banquet) | 12-oz. pkg. | 900 |
| CHICKEN PIE, frozen: | | |
| (Banquet) regular | 8-oz. pie | 540 |
| (Empire Kosher) | 8-oz. pie | 463 |
| (Stouffer's) | 10-oz. pie | 530 |
| (Swanson) regular | 8-oz. pie | 420 |
| CHICKEN PUFF, frozen (Durkee) | ½-oz. piece | 49 |
| CHICKEN SALAD (Carnation) | ¼ of 7½-oz. can | 94 |
| CHICKEN SOUP (See SOUP, Chicken) | | |
| CHICKEN SPREAD: | | |
| (Hormel) regular | 1 oz. | 60 |
| (Underwood) chunky | ½ of 4¾-oz. can | 63 |
| CHICKEN STEW, canned: | | |
| Regular: | | |
| (Libby's) with dumplings | 8 oz. | 194 |
| (Swanson) | 7⅜ oz. | 170 |
| Dietetic (Dia-Mel) | 8-oz. serving | 150 |
| CHICKEN STICKS, frozen (Country Pride) | 3 oz. | 233 |
| CHICKEN STOCK BASE (French's) | 1 tsp. | 8 |
| *CHICK-FIL-A:* | | |
| Brownie, fudge, with nuts | 2.8-oz. piece | 369 |
| Chicken, no bun | 3.6-oz. serving | 219 |
| Chicken nuggets, 8-pack | 4 oz. | 287 |
| Chicken salad: | | |
| Regular: | | |
| Cup | 3.4-oz. serving | 309 |
| Plate | 11.8-oz. serving | 475 |

| Food and Description | Measure or Quantity | Calories |
|---|---|---|
| Chargrilled, golden | 16.4-oz. serving | 126 |
| Sandwich, Chargrilled | 5½-oz. serving | 258 |
| Chicken sandwich, with bun: | | |
| Regular | 5¾-oz. serving | 360 |
| Deluxe Chargrilled, with lettuce & tomato | 7.15-oz. serving | 266 |
| Coleslaw | 3.7-oz. cup | 175 |
| *Icedream* | 4½-oz. serving | 134 |
| Pie, lemon | 4.1-oz. piece | 329 |
| Potato, *Waffle Potato Fries* | 3-oz. serving | 270 |
| Potato salad | 3.8-oz. serving | 198 |
| Salad, tossed: | | |
| Plain | 4½-oz. serving | 21 |
| With dressing: | | |
| Honey french | 6-oz. serving | 246 |
| Italian, light | 6-oz. serving | 46 |
| Thousand Island | 6-oz. serving | 231 |
| Soup, hearty breast of chicken, small | 8½-oz. serving | 152 |
| **CHICK'N QUICK,** frozen (Tyson): | | |
| Breast fillet | 3 oz. | 190 |
| Breast pattie | 3 oz. | 240 |
| *Chick'N Cheddar* | 3 oz. | 260 |
| Cordon bleu | 5 oz. | 310 |
| Kiev | 5 oz. | 430 |
| **CHICK PEA OR GARBANZO,** canned, solids & liq. (Allen's; Goya) | ½ cup | 110 |
| **CHILI OR CHILI CON CARNE:** | | |
| Canned, regular pack: | | |
| Beans only: | | |
| (Comstock) | ½ cup | 140 |
| (Hormel) | 5 oz. | 130 |
| (Hunt's) | 1 cup | 182 |
| (Van Camp) Mexican style | 1 cup | 250 |
| With beans: | | |
| (Gebhardt) hot | ½ of 15-oz. can | 470 |
| (Hormel) regular or hot | 7½-oz. serving | 310 |
| (Libby's) | 7½-oz. serving | 270 |
| (*Old El Paso*) | 1 cup | 349 |
| (Swanson) | 7¾-oz. serving | 310 |
| Without beans: | | |
| (Gebhardt) | ½ of 15-oz. can | 410 |
| (Hormel) regular or hot | 7½-oz. serving | 370 |
| (Libby's) | 7½ oz. | 390 |
| Canned, dietetic pack: | | |
| (Estee) with beans | 8-oz. serving | 370 |
| (Featherweight) with beans | 7½ oz. | 270 |
| Frozen (Stouffer's): | | |
| Regular, with beans | 8¾-oz. meal | 260 |

49

| Food and Description | Measure or Quantity | Calories |
|---|---|---|
| *Right Choice*, vegetarian | 9¾-oz. meal | 280 |
| **CHILI SAUCE:** | | |
| (Del Monte) | ¼ cup (2 oz.) | 70 |
| (El Molino) green, mild | 1 T. | 5 |
| (Heinz) | 1 T. | 17 |
| (La Victoria) | 1 T. | 3 |
| (Ortega) green, medium | 1 oz. | 7 |
| (Featherweight) Dietetic | 1 T. | 8 |
| **CHILI SEASONING MIX:** | | |
| *(Durkee) | 1 cup | 465 |
| (French's) *Chili-O*, plain | 1¾-oz. pkg. | 150 |
| (Lawry's) | 1.6-oz. pkg. | 143 |
| (McCormick) | 1.2-oz. pkg. | 106 |
| *CHOCO-DILE* (Hostess) | 2-oz. piece | 235 |
| **CHOCOLATE, BAKING:** | | |
| (Baker's): | | |
| Bitter or unsweetened | 1 oz. | 180 |
| Semi-sweet, chips | ½ cup | 207 |
| Sweetened, *German's* | 1 oz. | 158 |
| (Hershey's): | | |
| Bitter or unsweetened | 1 oz. | 190 |
| Sweetened: | | |
| Dark chips, regular or mini | 1 oz. | 151 |
| Milk, chips | 1 oz. | 150 |
| Semi-sweet, chips | 1 oz. | 147 |
| (Nestlé): | | |
| Bitter or unsweetened, *Choco-bake* | 1-oz. packet | 180 |
| Sweet or semi-sweet, morsels | 1 oz. | 150 |
| **CHOCOLATE ICE CREAM** (See ICE CREAM, Chocolate) | | |
| **CHOCOLATE SYRUP** (See SYRUP, Chocolate) | | |
| **CHOP SUEY,** frozen (Stouffer's) beef with rice | 12-oz. pkg. | 340 |
| ***CHOP SUEY SEASONING MIX** (Durkee) | 1¾ cups | 557 |
| **CHOWDER** (See SOUP, Chowder) | | |
| **CHOW MEIN:** | | |
| Canned: | | |
| (Chun King) Divider-Pak: | | |
| Beef | ¼ of pkg. | 91 |
| Chicken | ½ of 24-oz pkg. | 110 |
| Shrimp | ¼ of pkg. | 91 |
| (Hormel) Pork, *Short Orders* | 7½-oz. can | 140 |
| (La Choy): | | |
| Regular: | | |
| Beef | ¾ cup | 60 |
| Chicken | ¾ cup | 70 |
| Shrimp | ¾ cup | 45 |

| Food and Description | Measure or Quantity | Calories |
|---|---|---|
| *Bi-pack: | | |
| Beef | ¾ cup | 70 |
| Beef pepper oriental, chicken or shrimp | ¾ cup | 80 |
| Vegetable | ¾ cup | 50 |
| Frozen: | | |
| (Blue Star) *Dining Light,* chicken & rice | 11¼-oz. dinner | 233 |
| (Chun King) chicken | 13-oz. entree | 361 |
| (Empire Kosher) | ½ of 15-oz. pkg. | 97 |
| (La Choy): | | |
| Chicken | 12-oz. dinner | 260 |
| Shrimp | 12-oz. dinner | 220 |
| (Morton) chicken, light | 8-oz. entree | 210 |
| (Stouffer's) *Lean Cuisine,* with rice | 11¼-oz. serving | 250 |
| **CHOW MEIN SEASONING MIX** (Kikkoman) | 1⅛-oz. pkg. | 98 |
| *CHURCH'S FRIED CHICKEN:* | | |
| Chicken, fried: | | |
| Breast | 4.3-oz. piece | 278 |
| Leg | 2.9-oz. piece | 147 |
| Thigh | 4.2-oz. piece | 306 |
| Wing-breast | 4.8-oz. piece | 303 |
| Corn, with butter oil | 1 ear | 237 |
| French fried potatoes | 1 regular order | 138 |
| **CHUTNEY** (Major Grey's) | 1 T. | 53 |
| **CINNAMON, GROUND** (French's) | 1 tsp. | 6 |
| *CINNAMON TOAST CRUNCH,* cereal (General Mills) | ¾ cup | 120 |
| *CIRCUS FUN,* cereal (General Mills) | 1 cup | 110 |
| *CITRUS BERRY BLEND,* mix, dietetic (Sunkist) | 8 fl. oz. | 6 |
| **CITRUS COOLER DRINK,** canned (Hi-C) | 6 fl. oz. | 95 |
| **CLAM:** | | |
| Raw, all kinds, meat only | 1 cup (8 oz.) | 186 |
| Raw, soft, meat & liq. | 1 lb. (weighed in shell) | 142 |
| Canned (Doxsee): | | |
| Chopped, minced or whole: | | |
| Solids & liquid | ½ cup | 97 |
| Drained solids | ½ cup | 58 |
| Canned (Gorton's) minced, meat only | 1 can | 140 |
| Frozen: | | |
| (Gorton's) fried strips, crunchy | 1 package | 480 |
| (Howard Johnson's) | 5-oz. pkg. | 395 |
| (Mrs. Paul's) fried, light | 2½-oz. serving | 230 |

51

| Food and Description | Measure or Quantity | Calories |
|---|---|---|
| **CLAMATO COCKTAIL** (Mott's) | 6 fl. oz. | 80 |
| **CLAM JUICE** (Snow) | ½ cup | 15 |
| **CLARET WINE:** | | |
| (Gold Seal) | 3 fl. oz. | 82 |
| (Taylor) 12.5% alcohol | 3 fl. oz. | 72 |
| **CLORETS**, gum or mint | 1 piece | 6 |
| **CLUSTERS**, cereal | | |
| (General Mills) | ½ cup | 100 |
| **COCKTAIL** (see individual listings such as **DAIQUIRI, PIÑA COLADA**, etc.) | | |
| **COCOA:** | | |
| Dry, unsweetened: | | |
| (Hershey's) | 1 T. | 30 |
| (Sultana) | 1 T. | 30 |
| Mix, regular: | | |
| (Alba '66) instant, all flavors | 1 envelope | 60 |
| (Carnation) all flavors | 1-oz. pkg. | 110 |
| (Hershey's) instant | 3 T. | 81 |
| (Ovaltine) hot 'n rich | 1 oz. | 120 |
| *Swiss Miss*, regular or with mini marshmallows | 6 fl. oz. | 110 |
| Mix, dietetic: | | |
| (Carnation): | | |
| *70 Calorie* | ¾-oz. packet | 70 |
| *Sugar free | 6 fl. oz. | 50 |
| *(Featherweight) | 6 fl. oz. | 50 |
| *Swiss Miss*, instant, lite | 1 envelope | 70 |
| **COCOA KRISPIES**, cereal | | |
| (Kellogg's) | ¾ cup | 110 |
| **COCOA PUFFS**, cereal | | |
| (General Mills) | 1 oz. | 110 |
| **COCONUT:** | | |
| Fresh, meat only | 2″ × 2″ × ½″ piece | 156 |
| Grated or shredded, loosely packed | ½ cup | 225 |
| Dried: | | |
| (Baker's): | | |
| *Angel Flake* | ⅓ cup | 118 |
| Cookie | ⅓ cup | 186 |
| Premium shred | ⅓ cup | 138 |
| (Durkee) shredded | ¼ cup | 69 |
| **COCONUT, CREAM OF,** canned: | | |
| (Coco Lopez) | 1 T. | 60 |
| (Holland House) | 1 oz. | 81 |
| **COCO WHEATS**, cereal | 1 T. | 44 |
| **COD:** | | |
| Broiled | 3 oz. | 145 |
| Frozen: | | |
| (Frionor) *Norway Gourmet* | 4-oz. fillet | 70 |

| Food and Description | Measure or Quantity | Calories |
|---|---|---|
| (Van de Kamp's) *Today's Catch* | 4-oz. | 80 |
| **COD DINNER OR ENTREE,** frozen: | | |
| (Armour) *Dinner Classics,* almondine | 12-oz. dinner | 360 |
| (Frionor) *Norway Gourmet,* with dill sauce | 4½-oz. fillet | 80 |
| **COFFEE:** | | |
| Regular: | | |
| *Max-Pax; Maxwell House Electra Perk; Yuban, Yuban Electra Matic* | 6 fl. oz. | 2 |
| *Mellow Roast* | 6 fl.oz. | 8 |
| Decaffeinated: | | |
| *Brim,* regular or electric perk | 6 fl. oz. | 2 |
| *Brim,* freeze-dried; *Decafé; Nescafé* | 6 fl. oz. | 4 |
| *Sanka,* regular or electric perk | 6 fl. oz. | 2 |
| *Instant: | | |
| *Maxwell House; Taster's Choice* | 6 fl. oz. | 4 |
| *Mellow Roast* | 6 fl. oz. | 8 |
| *Sunrise* | 6 fl. oz. | 6 |
| *Mix (General Foods) International Coffee: | | |
| *Café Amaretto, Café Français* | 6 fl. oz. | 59 |
| *Café Vienna, Orange Cappuccino* | 6 fl. oz. | 65 |
| *Suisse Mocha* | 6 fl. oz. | 58 |
| **COFFEE CAKE** (See CAKE, Coffee) | | |
| **COFFEE LIQUEUR** (DeKuyper) | 1½ fl. oz. | 140 |
| **COFFEE SOUTHERN** | 1 fl. oz. | 79 |
| **COGNAC** (See DISTILLED LIQUOR) | | |
| **COLA SOFT DRINK** (See SOFT DRINK, Cola) | | |
| **COLD DUCK WINE** (Great Western) pink | 3 fl. oz. | 92 |
| **COLESLAW,** solids & liq., made with mayonnaise-type salad dressing | 1 cup | 119 |
| **\*COLESLAW MIX** (Libby's) *Super Slaw* | ½ cup | 240 |
| **COLLARDS:** | | |
| Leaves, cooked | ⅓ pkg. | 31 |
| Canned (Allen's) chopped, solids & liq. | ½ cup | 25 |
| Frozen: | | |
| (Birds Eye) chopped | ⅓ pkg. | 30 |
| (McKenzie) chopped | ⅓ pkg. | 25 |
| (Southland) chopped | ⅓ of 16-oz. pkg. | 25 |

| Food and Description | Measure or Quantity | Calories |
|---|---|---|
| **COMPLETE CEREAL** (Elam's) | 1 oz. | 109 |
| **CONCORD WINE:** | | |
| (Gold Seal) | 3 fl. oz. | 125 |
| (Pleasant Valley) red | 3 fl. oz. | 90 |
| **COOKIE, REGULAR:** | | |
| Almond Supreme (Pepperidge Farm) | 1 piece | 70 |
| Animal: | | |
| (Dixie Belle) | 1 piece | 8 |
| (Nabisco) *Barnum's Animals* | 1 piece | 12 |
| (Sunshine) | 1 piece | 8 |
| (Tom's) | ½ oz. | 62 |
| Apple N' Raisin (Archway) | 1 cookie | 120 |
| Apricot Raspberry (Pepperidge Farm) | 1 piece | 50 |
| Assortment: | | |
| (Nabisco) *Mayfair:* | | |
| Crown creme sandwich | 1 piece | 53 |
| Fancy shortbread biscuit | 1 piece | 22 |
| Filigree creme sandwich | 1 piece | 60 |
| *Mayfair* creme sandwich | 1 piece | 65 |
| Tea rose creme | 1 piece | 53 |
| (Pepperidge Farm): | | |
| Butter | 1 piece | 55 |
| *Champagne* | 1 piece | 32 |
| Chocolate lace & Pirouette | 1 piece | 37 |
| Seville | 1 piece | 55 |
| *Southport* | 1 piece | 75 |
| Blueberry (Pepperidge Farm) | 1 piece | 57 |
| *Blueberry Newtons* (Nabisco) | 1 piece | 73 |
| *Bordeaux* (Pepperidge Farm) | 1 piece | 33 |
| Brown edge wafer (Nabisco) | 1 piece | 28 |
| Brownie: | | |
| (Hostess) | 1.25-oz. piece | 157 |
| (Nabisco) *Almost Home* | 1¼-oz. piece | 160 |
| (Pepperidge Farm) chocolate nut | .4-oz. piece | 57 |
| *Brussels* (Pepperidge Farm) | 1 piece | 53 |
| *Brussels Mint* (Pepperidge Farm) | 1 piece | 67 |
| Butter (Sunshine) | 1 piece | 30 |
| *Cappucino* (Pepperidge Farm) | 1 piece | 53 |
| Caramel Patties (FFV) | 1 piece | 75 |
| *Chessman* (Pepperidge Farm) | 1 piece | 43 |
| Chocolate & chocolate-covered: | | |
| (Keebler) stripes | 1 piece | 50 |
| (Nabisco): | | |
| *Pinwheel,* cake | 1 piece | 130 |
| Snap | 1 piece | 19 |
| (Sunshine) nuggets | 1 piece | 23 |

54

| Food and Description | Measure or Quantity | Calories |
|---|---|---|
| Chocolate chip: | | |
| (Keebler) Rich 'n Chips | 1 piece | 80 |
| (Nabisco): | | |
| *Almost Home* | 1 piece | 65 |
| *Chips Ahoy!* | | |
| Regular | 1 piece | 47 |
| Chewy | 1 piece | 65 |
| Snaps | 1 piece | 22 |
| (Pepperidge Farm): | | |
| Regular | 1 piece | 50 |
| Chocolate | 1 piece | 53 |
| Mocha | 1 piece | 40 |
| (Sunshine): | | |
| *Chip-A-Roos* | 1 piece | 60 |
| *Chippy Chews* | 1 piece | 50 |
| (Tom's) | 1.7-oz. serving | 230 |
| Coconut fudge (FFV) | 1 piece | 80 |
| Date Nut Granola (Pepperidge Farm) | 1 piece | 53 |
| *Dinosaurs* (FFV) | 1 oz. | 130 |
| Dutch cocoa (Archway) | 1 piece | 110 |
| Fig bar: | | |
| (FFV) | 1 piece | 70 |
| (Nabisco) *Fig Newtons* | 1 piece | 50 |
| (Sunshine) Chewies | 1 piece | 50 |
| (Tom's) | 1.8-oz. serving | 170 |
| *Fruit Stick* (Nabisco) *Almost Home* | 1 piece | 70 |
| Gingerman (Pepperidge Farm) | 1 piece | 57 |
| Ginger Snap: | | |
| (Archway) | 1 piece | 25 |
| (FFV) | 1 oz. | 130 |
| (Nabisco) | 1 piece | 30 |
| (Sunshine) | 1 piece | 20 |
| Golden Fruit Raisin (Sunshine) | 1 piece | 70 |
| Hazelnut (Pepperidge Farm) | 1 piece | 57 |
| Ladyfinger | 3¼″ × 1⅜″ × 1⅛″ | 40 |
| *Lido* (Pepperidge Farm) | 1 piece | 95 |
| Macaroon, coconut (Nabisco) | 1 piece | 95 |
| *Mallow Puffs* (Sunshine) | 1 piece | 70 |
| Marshmallow: | | |
| (Nabisco): | | |
| *Mallomars* | 1 piece | 65 |
| Puffs, cocoa covered | 1 piece | 120 |
| Sandwich | 1 piece | 30 |
| *Twirls* cakes | 1 piece | 130 |
| (Planters) banana pie | 1 oz. | 127 |
| *Milano* (Pepperidge Farm) | 1 piece | 60 |
| *Mint Milano* (Pepperidge Farm) | 1 piece | 76 |
| Molasses: | | |
| (Archway) | 1 piece | 100 |

| Food and Description | Measure or Quantity | Calories |
|---|---|---|
| (Nabisco) *Pantry* | 1 piece | 65 |
| Molasses Crisp (Pepperidge Farm) | 1 piece | 33 |
| *Nilla* wafer (Nabisco) | 1 piece | 19 |
| Oatmeal: | | |
| (Archway): | | |
| Regular | 1 piece | 110 |
| Date filled | 1 piece | 100 |
| (FFV) bar | 1 piece | 70 |
| (Keebler) old fashioned | 1 piece | 80 |
| (Nabisco) *Bakers Bonus* | 1 piece | 65 |
| (Pepperidge Farm): | | |
| Irish | 1 piece | 47 |
| Raisin | 1 piece | 57 |
| (Sunshine) Country | 1 piece | 60 |
| *Orange Milano* (Pepperidge Farm) | 1 piece | 76 |
| *Orbits* (Sunshine) | 1 piece | 15 |
| Peach apricot bar (FFV) | 1 piece | 70 |
| Peanut & peanut butter (Nabisco): | | |
| *Almost Home* | 1 piece | 70 |
| *Nutter Butter*, sandwich | 1 piece | 70 |
| Pecan Sandies (Keebler) | 1 piece | 80 |
| Raisin: | | |
| (Nabisco) *Almost Home:* | | |
| Fudge chocolate chip | 1 piece | 65 |
| Iced applesauce | 1 piece | 70 |
| (Pepperidge Farm) bran | 1 piece | 53 |
| Raisin Bran (Pepperidge Farm) *Kitchen Hearth* | 1 piece | 53 |
| Raspberry filled (Archway) | 1 cookie | 105 |
| Rocky road (Archway) | 1 cookie | 130 |
| Sandwich: | | |
| (FFV) mint | 1 piece | 80 |
| (Keebler): | | |
| Fudge creme | 1 piece | 60 |
| *Pitter Patter* | 1 piece | 90 |
| (Nabisco): | | |
| Regular: | | |
| *Baronet* | 1 piece | 47 |
| *Gaity* | 1 piece | 50 |
| *Giggles* | 1 piece | 70 |
| *I Screams* | 1 piece | 75 |
| *Oreo*, regular | 1 piece | 47 |
| *Almost Home* | 1 piece | 140 |
| (Sunshine): | | |
| Regular, *Hydrox* | 1 piece | 50 |
| *Chips 'n Middles* | 1 piece | 70 |
| *Tru Blu* | 1 piece | 80 |
| Shortbread or shortcake: | | |

| Food and Description | Measure or Quantity | Calories |
|---|---|---|
| (Nabisco): | | |
| *Lorna Doone* | 1 piece | 35 |
| Pecan | 1 piece | 75 |
| (Pepperidge Farm) | 1 piece | 75 |
| *Social Tea,* biscuit (Nabisco) | 1 piece | 22 |
| Sprinkles (Sunshine) | 1 piece | 70 |
| Sugar cookie (Nabisco) rings, *Bakers Bonus* | 1 piece | 65 |
| Sugar wafer: | | |
| (Dutch Twin) any flavor | 1 piece | 36 |
| (Nabisco) *Biscos* | 1 piece | 19 |
| (Sunshine) | 1 piece | 45 |
| *Tahiti* (Pepperidge Farm) | 1 piece | 85 |
| Toy (Sunshine) | 1 piece | 12 |
| Vanilla wafer (FFV) | 1 piece | 130 |
| Waffle creme (Dutch Twin) | 1 piece | 45 |
| **COOKIE, DIETETIC** (Estee): | | |
| Chocolate chip, coconut or oatmeal raisin | 1 piece | 30 |
| Wafer, chocolate covered | 1 piece | 120 |
| *COOKIE CRISP,* cereal, any flavor | 1 cup | 110 |
| ***COOKIE DOUGH:*** | | |
| Refrigerated (Pillsbury): | | |
| Brownie, microwave, with chocolate chips | 1 piece | 180 |
| Oatmeal Raisin or peanut butter | 1 cookie | 70 |
| Frozen (Rich's): | | |
| Chocolate chip | 1 cookie | 138 |
| Oatmeal | 1 cookie | 125 |
| ***COOKIE MIX:*** | | |
| Regular: | | |
| Brownie: | | |
| (Betty Crocker): | | |
| Chocolate chip | ½₄ of pan | 130 |
| Frosted | ½₄ of pan | 160 |
| Fudge, family size | ½₄ of pan | 130 |
| Walnut | ½₄ of pan | 140 |
| (Pillsbury) fudge: | | |
| Regular | 2″ sq. (¹⁄₁₆ pkg.) | 150 |
| Microwave | ⅑ of pkg. | 190 |
| Ultimate, rocky road | 2″ sq. (¹⁄₁₆ of pkg.) | 170 |
| Chocolate chip: | | |
| (Betty Crocker) *Big Batch* | 1 cookie | 60 |
| (Duncan Hines) | ¹⁄₃₆ pkg. | 72 |
| (Nestlé) | 1 cookie | 60 |
| (Quaker) | 1 cookie | 75 |
| Fudge chip (Quaker) | 1 cookie | 75 |
| Macaroon, coconut (Betty Crocker) | ½₄ of pkg. | 80 |

57

| Food and Description | Measure or Quantity | Calories |
|---|---|---|
| Oatmeal (Quaker) | 1 cookie | 66 |
| Peanut butter (Duncan Hines) | 1/36 pkg. | 68 |
| Sugar: | | |
| (Betty Crocker) *Big Batch* | 1 cookie | 60 |
| (Duncan Hines) golden | 1 cookie | 59 |
| Dietetic (Estee) brownie | 2" × 2" sq. cookie | 45 |
| **COOKING SPRAY,** *Mazola No Stick* | 2-second spray | 8 |
| **CORN:** | | |
| Fresh, on the cob, boiled | 5" × 1¾" ear | 70 |
| Canned, regular pack, solids & liq.: | | |
| (Allen's) whole kernel | ½ cup | 80 |
| (Comstock) whole kernel | ½ cup | 90 |
| (Del Monte): | | |
| Cream style, golden | ½ cup | 95 |
| Whole kernel | ½ cup | 100 |
| (Green Giant): | | |
| Cream style | 4¼ oz. | 100 |
| Whole kernel, golden | 4¼ oz. | 80 |
| Whole kernel, *Mexicorn* | 3½ oz. | 80 |
| (Larsen) *Freshlike,* whole kernel, vacuum pack | ½ cup | 100 |
| (Libby's) cream style | ½ cup | 100 |
| (Stokely-Van Camp): | | |
| Cream style | ½ cup | 105 |
| Whole kernel, solids & liq. | ½ cup | 74 |
| Canned, dietetic pack, solids & liq.: | | |
| (Del Monte) No Salt Added | ½ cup | 70 |
| (Diet Delight) | ½ cup | 60 |
| (Larsen) *Fresh-Lite* | ½ cup | 80 |
| (S&W) *Nutradiet,* whole kernel, green label | ½ cup | 80 |
| Frozen: | | |
| (Birds Eye): | | |
| On the cob: | | |
| Regular | 4.4-oz. ear | 120 |
| *Little Ears* | 4.6-oz. ear | 126 |
| With butter sauce | ⅓ pkg. | 85 |
| (Frosty Acres): | | |
| On the cob | 1 whole ear | 120 |
| Kernels | 3.3 oz. | 80 |
| (Green Giant): | | |
| On the cob, regular: | | |
| *Nibbler* | 1 ear | 60 |
| Niblet Ear | 1 ear | 120 |
| Whole kernel, butter sauce, golden | 4 oz. | 100 |
| Whole kernel, *Niblets,* golden, polybag | ⅓ pkg. | 80 |

| Food and Description | Measure or Quantity | Calories |
|---|---|---|
| (Larsen): | | |
|   On the cob | 3″ piece (2.2 oz.) | 60 |
|   Kernels | 3.3 oz. | 80 |
| (Seabrook Farms): | | |
|   On the cob | 5″ ear | 140 |
|   Whole kernel | ⅓ pkg. | 97 |
| **CORNBREAD:** | | |
| Home recipe: | | |
|   Corn pone | 4 oz. | 231 |
|   Spoon bread | 4 oz. | 221 |
| *Mix: | | |
|   (Aunt Jemima) | ⅙ pkg. | 220 |
|   (Dromedary) | 2″ × 2″ piece | 130 |
|   (Pillsbury) *Ballard* | ⅛ of recipe | 140 |
| ***CORN DOGS,** frozen | | |
| (Hormel) | 1 piece | 220 |
| **CORNED BEEF:** | | |
| Cooked, boneless, medium fat | 4-oz. serving | 422 |
| Canned, regular pack: | | |
|   *Dinty Moore* (Hormel) | 2-oz. serving | 130 |
|   (Libby's) | ⅓ of 7-oz. can | 160 |
| Canned, dietetic (Featherweight) | | |
|   loaf | 2½-oz. serving | 90 |
| Packaged (Carl Buddig) sliced | 1-oz. slice | 40 |
| **CORNED BEEF HASH,** canned: | | |
| (Libby's) | ⅓ of 24-oz. can | 420 |
| *Mary Kitchen* (Hormel) | 7½-oz. serving | 360 |
| **CORNED BEEF HASH DINNER,** | | |
| frozen (Banquet) | 10-oz. dinner | 372 |
| **CORNED BEEF SPREAD** | | |
| (Underwood) | ½ of 4½-oz. can | 120 |
| **CORN FLAKE CRUMBS** | | |
| (Kellogg's) | ¼ cup | 110 |
| **CORN FLAKES,** cereal: | | |
| (General Mills) *Country* | 1 cup | 110 |
| (Kellogg's) regular | 1 cup | 110 |
| (Ralston Purina) regular | 1 cup | 110 |
| **CORN MEAL:** | | |
| Bolted (Aunt Jemima/Quaker) | 3 T. | 102 |
| Degermed | ¼ cup | 125 |
| Mix, bolted (Aunt Jemima) white | 1 cup | 392 |
| ***CORN POPS,*** cereal | | |
| (Kellogg's) | 1 cup | 110 |
| **CORN PUREE** (Larsen) | ½ cup | 100 |
| **CORNSTARCH** (Argo; Kingsford's; | | |
| Duryea) | 1 tsp. | 10 |
| **CORN SYRUP** (See SYRUP, Corn) | | |
| **COUGH DROP:** | | |
| (Beech-Nut) | 1 drop | 10 |

| Food and Description | Measure or Quantity | Calories |
|---|---|---|
| (Pine Bros.) | 1 drop | 10 |
| **COUNT CHOCULA,** cereal | | |
| (General Mills) | 1 oz. (1 cup) | 110 |
| **CRAB:** | | |
| Fresh, steamed: | | |
| Whole | ½ lb. | 101 |
| Meat only | 4 oz. | 105 |
| Canned, drained | 4 oz. | 115 |
| Frozen (Wakefield's) | 4 oz. | 96 |
| **CRAB APPLE,** flesh only | ¼ lb. | 71 |
| **CRAB APPLE JELLY** (Smucker's) | 1 T. | 53 |
| **CRAB AU GRATIN,** frozen | | |
| (Gorton's) *Light Recipe* | 1 package | 280 |
| **CRAB, DEVILED,** frozen | | |
| (Mrs. Paul's) breaded & fried, | | |
| regular | ½ of 6-oz. pkg. | 170 |
| **CRAB, IMITATION** (Louis Kemp) | | |
| *Crab Delights,* chunks, flakes or legs | 2 oz. | 60 |
| **CRAB IMPERIAL,** home recipe | 1 cup | 323 |
| **CRACKERS, PUFFS & CHIPS:** | | |
| Animal (FFV) | 1 oz. | 130 |
| Arrowroot biscuit (Nabisco) | 1 piece | 22 |
| Bacon-flavored thins (Nabisco) | 1 piece | 10 |
| *Bacon Nips* | 1 oz. | 147 |
| Bran wafer (Featherweight) | 1 piece | 13 |
| *Bravos* (Wise) | 1 oz. | 150 |
| *Bugles* (Tom's) | 1 oz. | 150 |
| Cafe (Sunshine) | 1 piece | 20 |
| Cheese flavored: | | |
| *American Heritage* (Sunshine): | | |
| Cheddar | 1 piece | 16 |
| Parmesan | 1 piece | 18 |
| Better Blue Thins (Nabisco) | 1 piece | 7 |
| Cheddar sticks (Flavor Tree) | 1 oz. | 160 |
| Cheese bites (Tom's) | 1½ oz. | 200 |
| *Cheese Doodles* (Wise): | | |
| Crunchy | 1 oz. | 160 |
| Puffed | 1 oz. | 150 |
| *Chee-Tos:* | | |
| Crunchy, regular | 1 oz. | 150 |
| Puffed balls or puffs | 1 oz. | 160 |
| *Cheez Balls* (Planters) | 1 oz. | 160 |
| *Cheez Curls* (Planters) | 1 oz. | 160 |
| *Cheeze-It* (Sunshine) | 1 piece | 6 |
| Corn Cheese (Tom's) crunchy | 1⅝ oz. | 280 |
| (Dixie Belle) | 1 piece | 6 |
| Nacho cheese cracker (Keebler) | 1 piece | 11 |
| *Nips* (Nabisco) | 1 piece | 5 |
| *Tid-Bit* (Nabisco) | 1 piece | 4 |

| Food and Description | Measure or Quantity | Calories |
|---|---|---|
| *Chicken in a Biskit* (Nabisco) | 1 piece | 10 |
| *Chipsters* (Nabisco) | 1 piece | 2 |
| *Club* cracker (Keebler) | 1 piece | 15 |
| Corn chips: | | |
| (Bachman) regular or BBQ | 1 oz. | 150 |
| *Dipsy Doodle* (Wise) | 1 oz. | 160 |
| (Featherweight) low sodium | 1 oz. | 170 |
| (Flavor Tree) | 1 oz. | 150 |
| *Fritos:* | | |
| Regular | 1 oz. | 150 |
| Chili cheese flavor | 1 oz. | 160 |
| *Korkers* (Nabisco) | 1 piece | 8 |
| (Laura Scudder's) | 1 oz. | 160 |
| (Tom's) regular | 1 oz. | 155 |
| Creme Wafer Stick (Nabisco) | 1 piece | 47 |
| Corn Stick (Flavor Tree) | 1 oz. | 160 |
| *Crown Pilot* (Nabisco) | 1 piece | 60 |
| *Diggers* (Nabisco) | 1 piece | 4 |
| English Water Biscuit | | |
| (Pepperidge Farm) | 1 piece | 17 |
| *Escort* (Nabisco) | 1 piece | 27 |
| French onion cracker (Nabisco) | 1 piece | 12 |
| *Goldfish* (Pepperidge Farm) | | |
| Tiny | 1 piece | 3 |
| Graham: | | |
| *Cinnamon Crisp* (Keebler) | 1 piece | 17 |
| (Dixie Belle) sugar-honey coated | 1 piece | 15 |
| *Flavor Kist* (Schulze and Burch) | | |
| sugar-honey coated | 1 piece | 57 |
| *Honey Maid* (Nabisco) | 1 piece | 30 |
| (Rokeach) | 8 pieces | 120 |
| (Sunshine) cinnamon | 1 piece | 17 |
| Graham, chocolate or cocoa-covered: | | |
| (Keebler) | 1 piece | 40 |
| (Nabisco) | 1 piece | 57 |
| *Great Crisps!* (Nabisco): | | |
| French onion | 1 piece | 10 |
| Nacho | 1 piece | 9 |
| Real bacon or sesame | 1 piece | 8 |
| *Hi Ho* (Sunshine) | 1 piece | 20 |
| *Meal Mates* (Nabisco) | 1 piece | 23 |
| Melba Toast (See MELBA TOAST) | | |
| Milk Lunch Biscuit (Keebler) | 1 piece | 27 |
| *Mucho Macho Nacho, Flavor Kist* | | |
| (Schulze and Burch) | 1 oz. | 121 |
| *Nachips* (Old El Paso) | 1 piece | 17 |
| Nacho Rings (Tom's) | 1 oz. | 160 |
| Ocean Crisp (FFV) | 1 piece | 60 |
| Onion rings (Wise) | 1 oz. | 130 |

| Food and Description | Measure or Quantity | Calories |
|---|---|---|
| Oyster: | | |
| (Dixie Belle) | 1 piece | 4 |
| (Keebler) *Zesta* | 1 piece | 2 |
| (Nabisco) *Dandy* or *Oysterettes* | 1 piece | 3 |
| (Sunshine) | 1 piece | 4 |
| Party (Estee) | ½ oz. | 70 |
| Party mix (Flavor Tree) | 1 oz. | 160 |
| Pizza Crunchies (Planters) | 1 oz. | 160 |
| *Ritz* (Nabisco) | 1 piece | 17 |
| *Roman Meal Wafer,* boxed | 1 piece | 11 |
| *Royal Lunch* (Nabisco) | 1 piece | 60 |
| Rusk, *Holland* (Nabisco) | 1 piece | 60 |
| Rye toast (Keebler) | 1 piece | 16 |
| *RyKrisp:* | | |
| Natural | 1 triple cracker | 20 |
| Seasoned | 1 triple cracker | 22 |
| Saltine: | | |
| (Dixie Belle) regular or unsalted | 1 piece | 12 |
| *Krispy* (Sunshine) | 1 piece | 12 |
| *Premium* (Nabisco) | 1 piece | 12 |
| (Rokeach) | 1 piece | 12 |
| *Zesta* (Keebler) | 1 piece | 12 |
| *Schooners* (FFV) whole wheat | ½ oz. | 70 |
| Sea Toast (Keebler) | 1 piece | 60 |
| Sesame: | | |
| *American Heritage* (Sunshine) | 1 piece | 17 |
| Butter flavored (Nabisco) | 1 piece | 17 |
| Chip (Flavor Tree) | 1 oz. | 150 |
| Crunch (Flavor Tree) | 1 oz. | 150 |
| (Estee) | ½ oz. | 70 |
| Stick (Flavor Tree): | | |
| Regular | 1 oz. | 150 |
| With bran or low sodium | 1 oz. | 160 |
| Toast (Keebler) | 1 piece | 16 |
| *Skittle Chips* (Nabisco) | 1 piece | 14 |
| Snackers (Ralston) | 1 piece | 17 |
| *Snackin Crisp* (Durkee) *D&C* | 1 oz. | 155 |
| Snacks Sticks (Pepperidge Farm): | | |
| Cheese | 1 piece | 17 |
| Lightly salted, pumpernickel, rye & sesame | 1 piece | 16 |
| *Sociables* (Nabisco) | 1 piece | 12 |
| Sour cream-onion stick (Flavor Tree) | 1 oz. | 150 |
| *Spirals* (Wise) | 1 oz. | 160 |
| Table Water Cracker (Carr's) small | 1 piece | 15 |
| Taco chip (Laura Scudder's) | 1 oz. | 150 |
| Tortilla chips: | | |

| Food and Description | Measure or Quantity | Calories |
|---|---|---|
| (Bachman) nacho, taco flavor or toasted | 1 oz. | 140 |
| *Doritos:* | | |
| Regular | 1 oz. | 140 |
| *Cool Ranch,* light | 1 oz. | 120 |
| *Salsa Rio* | 1 oz. | 140 |
| (Laura Scudder's) | 1 oz. | 140 |
| (Nabisco) regular and nacho | 1 piece | 11 |
| (Planters) | 1 oz. | 150 |
| (Tom's) | 1½ oz. | 210 |
| *Tostitos:* | | |
| Jalapeño & cheese | 1 oz. | 150 |
| Traditional | 1 oz. | 140 |
| *Town House Cracker* (Keebler) | 1 piece | 16 |
| *Triscuit* (Nabisco) | 1 piece | 20 |
| *Tuc* (Keebler) | 1 piece | 23 |
| *Twigs* (Nabisco) | 1 piece | 14 |
| *Uneeda Biscuit* (Nabisco) unsalted | 1 piece | 20 |
| Unsalted (Featherweight) | 2 sections (½ cracker) | 30 |
| *Waverly* (Nabisco) | 1 piece | 17 |
| Wheat (Pepperidge Farm) cracked or hearty | 1 piece | 25 |
| Wheatmeal Biscuit (Carr's) small | 1 piece | 42 |
| Wheat Nuts (Flavor Tree) | 1 oz. | 200 |
| Wheat Snack (Dixie Belle) | 1 piece | 9 |
| *Wheat Snax* (Estee) | 1 oz. | 110 |
| *Wheat Snaz* (Estee) | 1 oz. | 110 |
| *Wheatsworth* (Nabisco) | 1 piece | 14 |
| *Wheat Thins* (Nabisco) cheese | 1 piece | 9 |
| Wheat Toast (Keebler) | 1 piece | 15 |
| Wheat wafer (Featherweight) unsalted | 1 piece | 13 |
| **CRACKER CRUMBS,** graham: | | |
| (Nabisco) | 2 T. | 80 |
| (Sunshine) | ½ cup | 275 |
| **CRACKER MEAL** (Nabisco) | 2 T. | 50 |
| **CRANAPPLE JUICE** (Ocean Spray) canned: | | |
| Regular | 6 fl. oz. | 129 |
| Dietetic | 6 fl. oz. | 32 |
| **CRANBERRY,** fresh (Ocean Spray) | ½ cup | 26 |
| **CRANBERRY-APPLE JUICE COCKTAIL,** frozen (Welch's) | 6 fl. oz. | 120 |
| **CRANBERRY JUICE COCKTAIL:** | | |
| Canned (Ocean Spray): | | |
| Regular | 6 fl. oz. | 106 |
| Dietetic | 6 fl. oz. | 36 |
| *Frozen (Sunkist) | 6 fl. oz. | 110 |

| Food and Description | Measure or Quantity | Calories |
|---|---|---|
| **CRANBERRY-ORANGE RELISH** | | |
| (Ocean Spray) | 2 oz. | 104 |
| **CRANBERRY-RASPBERRY** | | |
| **SAUCE** (Ocean Spray) jellied | 2 oz. | 89 |
| **CRANBERRY SAUCE:** | | |
| Home recipe, sweetened, unstrained | 4 oz. | 202 |
| Canned (Ocean Spray): | | |
| Jellied | 2 oz. | 88 |
| Whole berry | 2 oz. | 89 |
| *CRANGRAPE* (Ocean Spray) | 6 fl. oz. | 108 |
| **CRANRASPBERRY** (Ocean Spray) | 6 fl. oz. | 110 |
| *CRANTASTIC JUICE DRINK,* | | |
| canned (Ocean Spray) | 6 fl. oz. | 110 |
| *CRAZY COW,* cereal (General Mills) | 1 cup | 110 |
| **CREAM:** | | |
| Half & half (Dairylea) | 1 fl. oz. | 40 |
| Heavy whipping (Dairylea) | 1 fl. oz. | 60 |
| Light, table or coffee: | | |
| (Johanna) 18% butterfat | 1 T. | 30 |
| (Sealtest) 16% butterfat | 1 T. | 26 |
| Light, whipping, 30% fat (Sealtest) | 1 T. | 45 |
| Sour: | | |
| (Dairylea) | 1 fl. oz. | 60 |
| (Johanna) | 1 T. (.5 oz.) | 31 |
| Sour, imitation (Pet) | 1 T. | 25 |
| Substitute (See CREAM SUBSTITUTE) | | |
| **CREAM PUFFS:** | | |
| Home recipe, custard filling | 3½″ × 2″ piece | 303 |
| Frozen (Rich's) chocolate | 1⅓-oz. piece | 146 |
| *CREAM OF RICE,* cereal | 1 oz. | 100 |
| *CREAMSICLE* (Popsicle Industries) | 2½-fl.-oz. piece | 80 |
| **CREAM SUBSTITUTE:** | | |
| *Coffee Mate* (Carnation) | 1 tsp. | 11 |
| *Coffee Rich* (Rich's) | ½ oz. | 22 |
| *Cremora* (Borden) | 1 tsp. | 12 |
| *Dairy Light* (Alba) | 2.8-oz. envelope | 10 |
| *Mocha Mix* (Presto Food Products) | 1 T. | 19 |
| *N-Rich* | 1 tsp. | 10 |
| (Pet) | 1 tsp. | 10 |
| *CREAM OF WHEAT,* cereal: | | |
| Regular | 1 oz. | 100 |
| *Instant | 1 oz. | 100 |
| *Mix'n Eat: | | |
| Regular | 1 packet | 100 |
| Apple & cinnamon | 1 packet | 130 |
| Maple & brown sugar | 1 packet | 130 |
| Quick | 1 T. | 40 |

| Food and Description | Measure or Quantity | Calories |
|---|---|---|
| **CREME DE BANANA LIQUEUR** | | |
| (Mr. Boston) | 1 fl. oz. | 93 |
| **CREME DE CACAO:** | | |
| (Hiram Walker) | 1 fl. oz. | 104 |
| (Mr. Boston): | | |
| Brown | 1 fl. oz. | 102 |
| White | 1 fl. oz. | 93 |
| **CREME DE CASSIS** (Mr. Boston) | 1 fl. oz. | 85 |
| **CREME DE MENTHE:** | | |
| (Bols) | 1 fl. oz. | 122 |
| (Mr. Boston): | | |
| Green | 1 fl. oz. | 109 |
| White | 1 fl. oz. | 97 |
| **CREME DE NOYAUX** (Mr. Boston) | 1 fl. oz. | 99 |
| **CREPE,** frozen: | | |
| (Mrs. Paul's): | | |
| Crab | 5½-oz. pkg. | 248 |
| Shrimp | 5½-oz. pkg. | 252 |
| (Stouffer's): | | |
| Chicken with mushroom sauce | 8¼-oz. pkg. | 390 |
| Spinach with cheddar cheese sauce | 9½-oz. pkg. | 415 |
| **CRISP RICE CEREAL:** | | |
| (Featherweight) low sodium | 1 cup | 110 |
| (Ralston Purina) | 1 cup | 110 |
| **CRISPY WHEATS'N RAISINS,** cereal (General Mills) | ¾ cup | 110 |
| **CROUTON:** | | |
| (Arnold): | | |
| Bavarian or English style | ½ oz. | 65 |
| French, Italian or Mexican style | ½ oz. | 66 |
| (Kellogg's) *Croutettes* | ⅔ cup | 70 |
| (Mrs. Culberson's) cheese & garlic or seasoned | .5 oz. | 60 |
| (Pepperidge Farm) | .5 oz. | 70 |
| **C-3PO'S,** cereal (Kellogg's) | ¾ cup | 110 |
| **CUCUMBER:** | | |
| Eaten with skin | 8-oz. cucumber | 32 |
| Pared | 7½" × 2" | 29 |
| Pared, | 3 slices (.9 oz.) | 4 |
| **CUMIN SEED** (French's) | 1 tsp. | 7 |
| **CUPCAKE:** | | |
| Regular (Hostess): | | |
| Chocolate | 1 cupcake | 170 |
| Orange | 1 cupcake | 150 |
| Frozen (Sara Lee) yellow | 1 cupcake | 190 |
| ***CUPCAKE MIX** (Flako) | 1 cupcake | 150 |
| **CUP O'NOODLES** (Nissin Foods): | | |
| Beef | 2½-oz. serving | 343 |

| Food and Description | Measure or Quantity | Calories |
|---|---|---|
| Beef onion | 2½-oz. serving | 323 |
| Chicken | 2½-oz. serving | 343 |
| Chicken, twin pack | 1.2-oz. serving | 155 |
| Shrimp | 2½-oz. serving | 336 |
| **CURAÇAO:** | | |
| (Bols) | 1 fl. oz. | 105 |
| (Hiram Walker) | 1 fl. oz. | 96 |
| **CURRANT, DRIED** (Del Monte) | | |
| Zante | ½ cup | 204 |
| **CURRANT JELLY,** sweetened | | |
| (Home Brands) | 1 T. | 50 |
| **CUSTARD:** | | |
| Canned (Thank You Brand) egg | ½ cup | 135 |
| Chilled, *Swiss Miss,* chocolate | | |
| or egg flavor | 4-oz. container | 150 |
| *Mix, dietetic (Featherweight) | ½ cup | 80 |
| *C. W. POST,* cereal: | | |
| Plain | ¼ cup | 130 |
| With raisins | ¼ cup | 120 |

# D

| Food and Description | Measure or Quantity | Calories |
|---|---|---|
| **DAIQUIRI COCKTAIL** | | |
| (Mr.Boston): | | |
| Regular | 3 fl. oz. | 99 |
| Strawberry | 3 fl. oz. | 111 |
| **\*DAIQUIRI COCKTAIL MIX:** | | |
| \*(Bar-Tender's) | 3½ fl. oz. | 177 |
| (Holland House): | | |
| Instant | .56 oz. | 65 |
| Liquid: | | |
| Regular | 1 oz. | 36 |
| Strawberry | 1 oz. | 31 |
| **DAIRY CRISP,** cereal (Pet) | ¼ cup | 120 |
| **DAIRY QUEEN/BRAZIER:** | | |
| Banana split | 13.5-oz. serving | 540 |
| *Brownie Delight,* hot fudge | 9.4-oz. serving | 600 |
| *Buster Bar* | 5¼-oz. piece | 460 |
| Chicken sandwich | 7.8-oz. sandwich | 670 |
| Cone: | | |
| Plain, any flavor, regular | 5-oz. cone | 240 |
| Dipped, chocolate, regular | 5½-oz. cone | 340 |
| *Dilly Bar* | 3-oz. piece | 210 |
| *Double Delight* | 9-oz. serving | 490 |
| *DQ Sandwich* | 2.1-oz. sandwich | 140 |
| Fish sandwich: | | |
| Plain | 6-oz. sandwich | 400 |
| With cheese | 6¼-oz. sandwich | 440 |
| Float | 14-oz. serving | 410 |
| Freeze, vanilla | 12-oz. serving | 500 |
| French fries: | | |
| Regular | 2½-oz. serving | 200 |
| Large | 4-oz. serving | 320 |
| Frozen dessert | 4-oz. serving | 180 |
| Hamburger: | | |
| Plain: | | |
| Single | 5.2-oz. burger | 360 |
| Double | 7.4-oz. burger | 530 |
| Triple | 9.6-oz. burger | 710 |
| With cheese: | | |
| Single | 5.7-oz. burger | 410 |

67

| Food and Description | Measure or Quantity | Calories |
|---|---|---|
| Double | 8.4-oz. burger | 650 |
| Triple | 10.63-oz. burger | 820 |
| Hot dog: | | |
| Regular: | | |
| Plain | 3.5-oz. serving | 280 |
| With cheese | 4-oz. serving | 330 |
| With chili | 4½-oz. serving | 320 |
| Super: | | |
| Plain | 6.2-oz. serving | 520 |
| With cheese | 6.9-oz. serving | 580 |
| With chili | 7.7-oz. serving | 570 |
| Malt, chocolate: | | |
| Large | 20¾-oz. serving | 1060 |
| Regular | 14¾-oz. serving | 760 |
| Small | 10¼-oz. serving | 520 |
| *Mr. Misty:* | | |
| Plain: | | |
| Large | 15½-oz. serving | 340 |
| Regular | 11.64-oz. serving | 250 |
| Small | 8¼-oz. serving | 190 |
| Kiss | 3.14-oz. serving | 70 |
| Float | 14.5-oz. serving | 390 |
| Freeze | 14.5-oz. serving | 500 |
| Onion rings | 3-oz. serving | 280 |
| Parfait | 10-oz. serving | 430 |
| *Peanut Butter Parfait* | 10¾-oz. serving | 750 |
| Shake, chocolate: | | |
| Large | 20¾-oz. serving | 990 |
| Regular | 14¾-oz. serving | 710 |
| Small | 10¼-oz. serving | 490 |
| Strawberry shortcake | 11-oz. serving | 540 |
| Sundae, chocolate: | | |
| Large | 8¾-oz. serving | 440 |
| Regular | 6¼-oz. serving | 310 |
| Small | 3¾-oz. serving | 190 |
| Tomato | ½ oz. | 4 |
| **DATE** (Dromedary): | | |
| Chopped | ¼ cup | 130 |
| Pitted | 5 dates | 100 |
| **DE CHAUNAC WINE** | | |
| (Great Western) 12% alcohol | 3 fl. oz. | 71 |
| *DELI'S,* frozen (Pepperidge Farm): | | |
| Mexican style | 4-oz. piece | 280 |
| Reuben in rye pastry | 4-oz. piece | 360 |
| Turkey, ham & cheese | 4-oz. piece | 270 |
| **DESSERT CUPS** (Hostess) | ¾-oz. piece | 62 |
| **DILL SEED** (French's) | 1 tsp. | 9 |
| *DING DONG* (Hostess) | 1 cake | 172 |

| Food and Description | Measure or Quantity | Calories |
|---|---|---|
| **DINNER,** frozen (See individual listings such as BEEF, CHICKEN, TURKEY, etc.) | | |
| **DIP:** | | |
| Acapulco (Ortega) with cheddar cheese | 1 oz. | 64 |
| Avocado (Nalley's) | 1 oz. | 114 |
| Bacon & horseradish (Kraft) | 1 T. | 30 |
| Bacon & onion (Nalley's) | 1 oz. | 113 |
| Barbecue (Nalley's) | 1 oz. | 114 |
| Blue cheese: | | |
| (Dean) tang | 1 oz. | 61 |
| (Nalley's) | 1 oz. | 110 |
| Chili (La Victoria) | 1 T. | 6 |
| Clam (Nalley's) | 1 oz. | 101 |
| Cucumber & onion (Breakstone) | 1 oz. | 50 |
| Guacamole (Calavo) | 1 oz. | 55 |
| Jalapeño: | | |
| *Fritos* | 1 oz. | 34 |
| (Hain) natural | 1 oz. | 40 |
| (Wise) | 1 T. | 12 |
| Onion (Thank You Brand) | 1 T. | 45 |
| Onion bean (Hain) natural | 1 oz. | 41 |
| Picante sauce (Wise) | 1 T. | 6 |
| Taco (Thank You Brand) | 1 T. | 44 |
| **DIP 'UM SAUCE,** canned (French's): | | |
| BBQ | 1 T. | 22 |
| Hot mustard | 1 T. | 35 |
| Sweet 'n sour | 1 T. | 40 |
| **DISTILLED LIQUOR,** any brand: | | |
| 80 proof | 1 fl. oz. | 65 |
| 86 proof | 1 fl. oz. | 70 |
| 90 proof | 1 fl. oz. | 74 |
| 94 proof | 1 fl. oz. | 77 |
| 100 proof | 1 fl. oz. | 83 |
| **DONUTZ,** cereal (General Mills) | 1 cup | 120 |
| **DOUGHNUT** (See also *WINCHELL'S*): | | |
| Regular: | | |
| (Hostess): | | |
| Chocolate coated | 1-oz. piece | 130 |
| Cinnamon | 1-oz. piece | 110 |
| *Donettes,* powdered | 1 piece | 40 |
| Old fashioned, plain | 1.5-oz. piece | 180 |
| Powdered | 1-oz. piece | 110 |
| (Dolly Madison): | | |
| Regular: | | |
| Plain or coconut crunch | 1¼-oz. piece | 140 |
| Chocolate coated | 1¼-oz. piece | 150 |

| Food and Description | Measure or Quantity | Calories |
|---|---|---|
| Dunkin' Stix | 1⅜-oz. piece | 210 |
| Gems: | | |
| Chocolate coated | .5-oz. piece | 65 |
| Powdered sugar | .5-oz. piece | 10 |
| Jumbo: | | |
| Plain or cinnamon sugar | 1.6-oz. piece | 190 |
| Sugar | 1.7-oz. piece | 210 |
| Old fashioned: | | |
| Chocolate glazed or powdered sugar | 2.2-oz. piece | 260 |
| Cinnamon chip, glazed or orange crush | 2.2-oz. piece | 280 |
| White iced | 2.2-oz. piece | 300 |
| Frozen (Morton): | | |
| Regular: | | |
| Boston creme | 2-oz. piece | 180 |
| Chocolate iced | 1.5-oz. piece | 150 |
| Jelly | 1.8-oz. piece | 180 |
| Donut Holes | ⅓ of 7¾-oz. pkg. | 160 |
| Morning Light, jelly | 2.6-oz. piece | 250 |
| DRAMBUIE (Hiram Walker) | 1 fl. oz. | 110 |
| DRUMSTICK, frozen: | | |
| Ice cream, in a cone: | | |
| Topped with peanuts | 1 piece | 181 |
| Topped with peanuts & cone bisque | 1 piece | 168 |
| Ice milk, in a cone: | | |
| Topped with peanuts | 1 piece | 163 |
| Topped with peanuts & cone bisque | 1 piece | 150 |
| DULCITO, frozen (Hormel) apple | 4 oz. | 290 |
| DUMPLINGS, canned, dietetic (Dia-Mel) | 8-oz. serving | 160 |

# E

| Food and Description | Measure or Quantity | Calories |
|---|---|---|
| **ECLAIR:** | | |
| Home recipe, with custard filling and chocolate icing | 4-oz. piece | 271 |
| Frozen (Rich's) chocolate | 1 piece | 196 |
| **EEL,** smoked, meat only | 4 oz. | 374 |
| **EGG, CHICKEN:** | | |
| Raw: | | |
| White only | 1 large egg | 17 |
| Yolk only | 1 large egg | 59 |
| Boiled | 1 large egg | 81 |
| Fried in butter | 1 large egg | 99 |
| Omelet, mixed with milk & cooked in fat | 1 large egg | 107 |
| Poached | 1 large egg | 78 |
| Scrambled, mixed with milk & cooked in fat | 1 large egg | 111 |
| **EGG DINNER OR ENTREE,** frozen (Swanson): | | |
| Omelet, Spanish style | 7¾-oz. meal | 250 |
| Scrambled, with sausage & potatoes | 6¼-oz. meal | 410 |
| ***EGG FOO YUNG,** dinner: | | |
| (Chun King) stir fry | 5 oz. | 138 |
| (La Choy) | 1 patty plus ¼ cup sauce | 164 |
| **EGG MIX** (Durkee): | | |
| Omelet: | | |
| *With bacon | ½ pkg. | 310 |
| *Puffy | ½ pkg. | 302 |
| Scrambled: | | |
| Plain | .8-oz. pkg. | 124 |
| With bacon | 1.3-oz. pkg. | 181 |
| **EGG NOG,** dairy: | | |
| (Borden) | ½ cup | 160 |
| (Johanna) | ½ cup | 195 |
| **EGG NOG COCKTAIL** | | |
| (Mr. Boston) 15% alcohol | 3 fl. oz. | 177 |
| **EGGPLANT:** | | |
| Boiled, drained | 4 oz. | 22 |

71

| Food and Description | Measure or Quantity | Calories |
|---|---|---|
| Frozen: | | |
| (Buitoni) parmigiana | 5 oz. | 168 |
| (Celentano) rollettes | 11-oz. pkg. | 420 |
| (Mrs. Paul's): | | |
| Parmesan | 5½-oz. serving | 270 |
| Sticks, breaded & fried | 3½-oz. serving | 240 |
| (Weight Watchers) Parmesan | 13-oz. pkg. | 285 |
| **EGG ROLL,** frozen: | | |
| (Chun King): | | |
| Chicken | 3.5-oz. piece | 210 |
| Meat & shrimp | 3.5-oz. piece | 214 |
| Shrimp | 3.5-oz. piece | 189 |
| (La Choy): | | |
| Almond chicken, entree | 2 egg rolls | 450 |
| Beef & broccoli, entree | 2 egg rolls | 380 |
| Chicken | .5-oz. piece | 30 |
| Lobster | 3-oz. piece | 180 |
| Shrimp | .5-oz. piece | 27 |
| **EGG ROLL DINNER,** frozen (Van de Kamp's) Cantonese | 10½-oz. serving | 560 |
| **EGG SUBSTITUTE:** | | |
| *Egg Magic* (Featherweight) | ½ envelope | 60 |
| *Scramblers* (Morningstar Farms) | 1 egg substitute | 35 |
| *Second Nature* (Avoset) | 3 T. | 42 |
| **EL POLLO LOCO,** restaurant: | | |
| Beans | 3½-oz. serving | 110 |
| Chicken | 2 pieces (4.8-oz. edible portion) | 310 |
| Coleslaw | 2.8-oz. serving | 80 |
| Combo meal | 16-oz. serving | 720 |
| Corn | 3.3-oz. serving | 110 |
| Dole Whip | 4½-oz. serving | 90 |
| Potato Salad | 4.3-oz. serving | 140 |
| Rice | 2½-oz. serving | 100 |
| Salsa | 1.8-oz. serving | 10 |
| Tortilla: | | |
| Corn | 3.3-oz. serving | 210 |
| Flour | 3.3-oz. serving | 280 |
| **ENCHILADA OR ENCHILADA DINNER,** frozen: | | |
| Beef: | | |
| (Banquet): | | |
| Dinner | 12-oz. meal | 497 |
| Entree | 2-lb. pkg | 1056 |
| (Fred's) *Marquez* | 7½-oz. serving | 304 |
| (Green Giant) Sonora style | 12-oz. entree | 700 |
| (Hormel) | 1 enchilada | 140 |
| (Morton) | 11-oz. dinner | 280 |

72

| Food and Description | Measure or Quantity | Calories |
|---|---|---|
| (Patio) | 13¼-oz. meal | 514 |
| (Stouffer's) & bean, *Lean Cuisine* | 9¼-oz. meal | 280 |
| (Van de Kamp's): | | |
| Dinner, regular | 12-oz. dinner | 390 |
| Entree, shredded | 5½-oz. serving | 180 |
| Cheese: | | |
| (Banquet) | 12-oz. dinner | 543 |
| (Patio) | 12¼-oz. meal | 378 |
| (Van de Kamp's) | 12-oz. dinner | 450 |
| Chicken (Van de Kamp's) | 7½-oz. pkg. | 250 |
| **ENCHILADA SAUCE:** | | |
| Canned: | | |
| (Del Monte) hot or mild | ½ cup | 45 |
| (El Molino) hot | 1 T. | 8 |
| (La Victoria) | 1 T. | 5 |
| *Old El Paso*, hot | ¼ cup | 27 |
| *Mix (Durkee) | ½ cup | 29 |
| **ENCHILADA SEASONING MIX** | | |
| (Lawry's) | 1.6-oz. pkg. | 152 |
| **ENDIVE, CURLY OR ESCAROLE,** cut | ½ cup | 7 |
| ***ESPRESSO COFFEE LIQUEUR*** | 1 fl. oz. | 104 |

# F

| Food and Description | Measure or Quantity | Calories |
|---|---|---|
| **FAJITA SEASONING MIX** (Lawry's) | 1.3-oz. pkg. | 63 |
| **FARINA:** | | |
| (Hi-O) dry, regular | 1 T. | 40 |
| *Malt-O-Meal,* dry: | | |
| Regular | 1 oz. | 96 |
| Quick cooking | 1 oz. | 100 |
| *(Pillsbury) made with water and salt | ⅔ cup | 80 |
| **FAT, COOKING:** | | |
| *Crisco:* | | |
| Regular | 1 T. | 110 |
| Butter flavor | 1 T. | 126 |
| (Rokeach) neutral nyafat | 1 T. | 99 |
| *Spry* | 1 T. | 94 |
| **FENNEL SEED** (French's) | 1 tsp. | 8 |
| **FETTUCINI ALFREDO,** frozen | | |
| (Stouffer's) | ½ of 10-oz. pkg. | 270 |
| **FIBER ONE,** cereal | | |
| (General MIlls) | ½ cup | 60 |
| **FIG:** | | |
| Small | 1½" fig | 30 |
| Canned, regular pack (Del Monte) | | |
| whole, solids & liq. | ½ cup | 100 |
| Dried (Sun-Maid), Calimyrna | ½ cup | 250 |
| **FIG JUICE** (Sunsweet) | 6 fl. oz. | 120 |
| **FIGURINES** (Pillsbury) all flavors | 1 bar | 100 |
| **FILBERT:** | | |
| Shelled | 1 oz. | 180 |
| (Fisher) oil dipped, salted | ½ cup | 360 |
| **FISH CAKE,** frozen (Mrs. Paul's): | | |
| Breaded & fried | 2-oz. piece | 110 |
| Thins, breaded & fried | ½ of 10-oz. pkg. | 300 |
| **FISH & CHIPS,** frozen: | | |
| (Gorton's) | 1 pkg. | 1350 |
| (Swanson): | | |
| Regular | 5½-oz. entree | 320 |
| *Hungry Man* | 14¾-oz. dinner | 770 |
| (Van de Kamp's) batter dipped, | | |
| french fried | 7-oz. pkg. | 440 |

| Food and Description | Measure or Quantity | Calories |
|---|---|---|
| **FISH DINNER**, frozen: | | |
| (Banquet) | 8¾-oz. dinner | 445 |
| (Morton) | 10-oz. dinner | 367 |
| (Mrs. Paul's) Parmesan | ½ of 10-oz. pkg. | 220 |
| (Stouffer's) *Lean Cuisine*, Florentine | 9-oz. pkg. | 230 |
| (Weight Watchers): | | |
| Au gratin | 9½-oz. meal | 200 |
| Oven fried | 6¾-oz. meal | 220 |
| **FISH FILLET**, frozen: | | |
| (Frionor) *Bunch O' Crunch*, breaded | 1 piece | 140 |
| (Gorton's): | | |
| Regular, crunchy | 1 piece | 175 |
| *Light Recipe*, tempura batter | 1 piece | 190 |
| (Mrs. Paul's): | | |
| Batter fried, crunchy | 2¼-oz. piece | 155 |
| Breaded & fried, light & natural | 1 piece | 290 |
| (Van de Kamp's): | | |
| Batter dipped, french fried | 3-oz. piece | 180 |
| Country seasoned | 2-oz. piece | 200 |
| **FISH KABOBS**, frozen: | | |
| (Mrs. Paul's) light batter | ⅓ pkg. | 200 |
| (Van de Kamp's) batter dipped, french fried | 4-oz. piece | 240 |
| **FISH NUGGET**, frozen (Frionor) *Bunch O' Crunch*, breaded | 1 piece | 40 |
| **FISH SANDWICH**, frozen (Frionor) *Bunch O' Crunch*, microwave | 5-oz. sandwich | 320 |
| **FISH SEASONING** (Featherweight) | ¼ tsp. | <1 |
| **FISH STICKS**, frozen: | | |
| (Frionor) *Bunch O' Crunch*, breaded | .7-oz. piece | 58 |
| (Gorton's) potato crisp | 1 piece | 60 |
| (Mrs. Paul's): | | |
| Batter fried | 1 piece | 69 |
| Breaded & fried | 1 piece | 43 |
| (Van de Kamp's) batter dipped, french fried | 1-oz. piece | 55 |
| ***FIT'N FROSTY*** (Alba '77): | | |
| Chocolate or marshmallow flavor | 1 envelope | 70 |
| Strawberry | 1 envelope | 74 |
| Vanilla | 1 envelope | 69 |
| *****FIVE ALIVE*** (Snow Crop) | 6 fl. oz. | 85 |
| **FLOUNDER:** | | |
| Baked | 4 oz. | 229 |
| Frozen: | | |
| (Frionor) *Norway Gourmet* | 4-oz. fillet | 60 |
| (Gorton's) *Fishmarket Fresh* | 4 oz. | 90 |

| Food and Description | Measure or Quantity | Calories |
|---|---|---|
| (Mrs. Paul's) fillets, breaded & fried, crispy, crunchy | 2-oz. piece | 140 |
| **FLOUNDER DINNER OR ENTREE,** frozen (Le Menu) | 10½-oz. dinner | 340 |
| **FLOUR:** | | |
| (Aunt Jemima) self-rising | ¼ cup | 109 |
| *Ballard,* self-rising | ¼ cup | 100 |
| *Bisquick* (Betty Crocker) | ¼ cup | 115 |
| (Elam's): | | |
| Brown rice, whole grain | ¼ cup | 146 |
| Buckwheat, pure | ¼ cup | 92 |
| Pastry | 1 oz. | 102 |
| Rye, whole grain | ¼ cup | 89 |
| Soy | 1 oz. | 98 |
| *Gold Medal* (Betty Crocker) all-purpose or high protein | ¼ cup | 100 |
| *La Pina* | ¼ cup | 100 |
| *Pillsbury's Best:* | | |
| All-purpose or rye, medium | ¼ cup | 100 |
| Sauce & gravy | 2 T. | 50 |
| Self-rising | ¼ cup | 95 |
| *Presto,* self-rising | ¼ cup | 98 |
| *Wondra* | ¼ cup | 100 |
| **FOOD STICKS** (Pillsbury) chocolate | 1 piece | 45 |
| **FRANKEN\*BERRY,** cereal (General Mills) | 1 cup | 110 |
| **FRANKFURTER:** | | |
| (Eckrich): | | |
| Beef, or meat | 1.6-oz. frankfurter | 150 |
| Beef or meat, jumbo | 2-oz. frankfurter | 190 |
| Meat | 1.2-oz. frankfurter | 120 |
| (Empire Kosher): | | |
| Chicken | 2-oz. frankfurter | 106 |
| Turkey | 2-oz. frankfurter | 107 |
| *Hebrew National:* | | |
| Beef | 1.7-oz. frankfurter | 149 |
| Natural casing | 2-oz. frankfurter | 175 |
| (Hormel): | | |
| Beef | 1.6-oz. frankfurter | 139 |
| *Range Brand, Wrangler,* smoked | 1 frankfurter | 160 |
| (Hygrade) beef, *Ball Park* | 2-oz. frankfurter | 169 |
| (Louis Rich) turkey | 1.5-oz. frankfurter | 95 |
| (Ohse): | | |
| Regular, beef | 1-oz. frankfurter | 85 |
| Wiener: | | |
| Regular | 1-oz. frankfurter | 90 |
| Chicken | 1-oz. frankfurter | 85 |
| (Oscar Mayer): | | |
| Bacon & cheddar | 1.6-oz. frankfurter | 139 |

| Food and Description | Measure or Quantity | Calories |
|---|---|---|
| Beef | 1.6-oz. frankfurter | 143 |
| Cheese | 1.6-oz. frankfurter | 144 |
| Little Wiener | 2″ frankfurter | 28 |
| Wiener | 1.6-oz. frankfurter | 144 |
| **FRANKS-N-BLANKETS,** frozen (Durkee) | 1 piece | 45 |
| **FRENCH TOAST,** frozen: | | |
| (Aunt Jemima): | | |
| Regular | 1 slice | 85 |
| Cinnamon swirl | 1 slice | 97 |
| (Swanson) with sausage, plain | 6½-oz. meal | 450 |
| **FRITTERS,** frozen (Mrs. Paul's): | | |
| Apple | 2-oz. piece | 125 |
| Clam | 1.9-oz. piece | 131 |
| Corn | 2-oz. piece | 73 |
| Shrimp | ½ of 7¾-oz. pkg. | 242 |
| **FROOT LOOPS,** cereal (Kellogg's) | 1 cup | 110 |
| **FROSTED RICE,** cereal (Kellogg's) | 1 cup | 110 |
| **FROSTEE** (Borden): | | |
| Chocolate | 1 cup | 200 |
| Strawberry | 1 cup | 180 |
| **FROSTS** (Libby's): | | |
| Dry: | | |
| Banana | .5 oz. | 50 |
| Orange, strawberry or pineapple | .5 oz. | 60 |
| Liquid: | | |
| Banana | 7 fl. oz. | 120 |
| Orange or strawberry | 8 fl. oz. | 120 |
| **FROZEN DESSERT,** dietetic (See also *TOFUTTI*): | | |
| (Baskin-Robbins): | | |
| *Low, Lite 'N Luscious* | ½ cup (4 fl. oz.) | 80–100 |
| *Special Diet* | 1 scoop (2½ fl. oz.) | 90 |
| *Eskimo,* bar, chocolate covered | 2½-fl.-oz. bar | 110 |
| *Mocha Mix* (Presto Food Products) | | |
| Bar, vanilla, chocolate covered | 4-fl.-oz. piece | 230 |
| Bulk: | | |
| Dutch chocolate, strawberry swirl or vanilla | 4 fl. oz. | 140 |
| Heavenly hash | 4 fl. oz. | 160 |
| Toasted almond | 4 fl. oz. | 150 |
| (SugarLo) all flavors | ¼ pt. | 135 |
| **FRUIT BARS** (General Mills) *Fruit Corners* | 1 bar | 90 |
| **FRUIT BITS,** dried (Sun-Maid) | 1 oz. | 90 |
| **FRUIT COCKTAIL:** | | |
| Canned, regular pack, solids & liq.: | | |
| (Del Monte) regular or chunky | ½ cup | 94 |

| Food and Description | Measure or Quantity | Calories |
|---|---|---|
| (Libby's) | ½ cup | 101 |
| (Stokely-Van Camp) | ½ cup | 95 |
| Canned, dietetic or low calorie, solids & liq.: | | |
| (Del Monte) Lite | ½ cup | 58 |
| (Diet Delight): | | |
| Syrup pack | ½ cup | 50 |
| Water pack | ½ cup | 40 |
| (Featherweight): | | |
| Juice pack | ½ cup | 50 |
| Water pack | ½ cup | 40 |
| (Libby's) water pack | ½ cup | 50 |
| (S&W) *Nutradiet:* | | |
| Juice pack | ½ cup | 50 |
| Water pack | ½ cup | 40 |
| **FRUIT COMPOTE** (Rokeach) | ½ cup | 120 |
| ***FRUIT COUNTRY*** (Comstock): | | |
| Apple or blueberry | ¼ pkg. | 160 |
| Cherry | ¼ pkg. | 180 |
| **FRUIT CUP** (Del Monte): | | |
| Mixed fruits | 5-oz. container | 110 |
| Peaches, diced | 5-oz. container | 116 |
| **FRUIT, MIXED:** | | |
| Canned (Del Monte) lite, chunky | ½ cup | 58 |
| Frozen (Birds Eye) quick thaw | 5-oz. serving | 150 |
| ***FRUIT & FIBER CEREAL*** (Post) | ½ cup | 103 |
| **FRUIT JUICE,** canned (Sun-Maid) | 6 fl. oz. | 100 |
| **FRUIT 'N APPLE JUICE** (Tree Top) | 6 fl. oz. | 90 |
| **FRUIT 'N GRAPE JUICE** (Tree Top): | | |
| Canned | 6 fl. oz. | 100 |
| *Frozen | 6 fl. oz. | 110 |
| ***FRUIT 'N JUICE BAR*** (Dole) | 2½-fl.-oz. bar | 70 |
| **FRUIT & NUT MIX** (Carnation): | | |
| All fruit | .9-oz. pouch | 80 |
| Deluxe trail mix or raisins & nuts | .9-oz. pouch | 130 |
| Tropical fruit & nuts | .9-oz. pouch | 100 |
| **FRUIT PUNCH:** | | |
| Canned: | | |
| *Capri Sun* | 6¾ fl. oz. | 102 |
| (Hi-C) | 6 fl. oz. | 96 |
| (Lincoln) | 6 fl. oz. | 90 |
| Chilled: | | |
| *Five Alive* (Snow Crop) | 6 fl. oz. | 87 |
| (Sunkist) | 8.45 fl. oz. | 140 |
| *Frozen, *Five Alive* (Snow Crop) | 6 fl. oz. | 87 |
| **FRUIT ROLL:** | | |
| (Betty Crocker) | 1 piece | 50 |
| (Flavor Tree) | ¾-oz. roll | 80 |

| Food and Description | Measure or Quantity | Calories |
|---|---|---|
| Fruit Roll-Ups, Fruit Corners: | | |
| Apple, apricot, cherry, grape or strawberry | .5-oz. roll | 50 |
| Fruit punch | .5-oz. roll | 60 |
| (Sunkist) | ½-oz. piece | 50 |
| **FRUIT SALAD:** | | |
| Canned, regular pack: | | |
| (Del Monte) fruits for salad | ½ cup | 93 |
| (Libby's) | ½ cup | 99 |
| Canned, dietetic or low calorie: | | |
| (Diet Delight) | ½ cup | 60 |
| (Featherweight): | | |
| Juice pack | ½ cup | 50 |
| Water pack | ½ cup | 40 |
| (S&W) *Nutradiet:* | | |
| Juice pack | ½ cup | 60 |
| Water pack | ½ cup | 35 |
| **FRUIT SQUARES,** frozen (Pepperidge Farm) | 2½-oz. piece | 230 |
| **FRUIT WRINKLES,** *Fruit Corners* | 1 pouch | 100 |
| **FUDGSICLE** (Popsicle Industries) | 2½-fl.-oz. bar | 100 |

# G

| Food and Description | Measure or Quantity | Calories |
|---|---|---|
| **GARLIC:** | | |
| Flakes (Gilroy) | 1 tsp. | 5 |
| Powder (French's) with parsley | 1 tsp. | 12 |
| Salt (Lawry's) | 1 tsp. | 4 |
| Spread (Lawry's) concentrate | 1 T. | 15 |
| **GEFILTE FISH,** canned: | | |
| (Mother's): | | |
| Jellied, old world | 4-oz. serving | 70 |
| Jellied, white fish & pike | 4-oz. serving | 60 |
| In liquid broth | 4-oz. serving | 70 |
| (Rokeach): | | |
| Natural Broth | 2-oz. serving | 46 |
| Old Vienna: | | |
| Regular | 2-oz. serving | 52 |
| Jelled | 2-oz. serving | 54 |
| **GELATIN,** dry, *Carmel Kosher* | 7-gram envelope | 30 |
| ***GELATIN DESSERT MIX:** | | |
| Regular: | | |
| *Carmel Kosher,* all flavors | ½ cup | 80 |
| (Jell-O) all flavors | ½ cup | 81 |
| Dietetic: | | |
| *Carmel Kosher* | ½ cup | 8 |
| (D-Zerta) all flavors | ½ cup | 6 |
| (Featherweight) artificially | | |
| sweetened or regular | ½ cup | 10 |
| *(Royal) | ½ cup | 12 |
| **GELATIN, DRINKING** (Knox) | | |
| orange | 1 envelope | 39 |
| **GERMAN STYLE DINNER,** frozen | | |
| (Swanson) | 11¾-oz. dinner | 370 |
| **GIN, SLOE:** | | |
| (Bols) | 1 fl. oz. | 85 |
| (DeKuyper) | 1 fl. oz. | 70 |
| (Mr. Boston) | 1 fl. oz. | 68 |
| **GINGER,** powder (French's) | 1 tsp. | 6 |
| ***GINGERBREAD:** | | |
| Home recipe (USDA) | 1.9-oz. piece | 174 |
| Mix: | | |
| (Betty Crocker) | ⅑ of cake | 210 |

| Food and Description | Measure or Quantity | Calories |
|---|---|---|
| (Dromedary) | 2″ × 2″ square | 100 |
| (Pillsbury) | 3″ square | 190 |
| **GOLDEN GRAHAMS,** cereal | | |
| (General Mills) | ¾ cup | 110 |
| **GOOBER GRAPE** (Smucker's) | 1 T. | 90 |
| **GOOD HUMOR** (See ICE CREAM) | | |
| **GOOD N' PUDDIN** | | |
| (Popsicle Industries) all flavors | 2⅓-fl.-oz. bar | 170 |
| **GOOSE,** roasted, meat & skin | 4 oz. | 500 |
| **GRAHAM CRAKOS,** cereal | | |
| (Kellogg's) | 1 cup | 110 |
| **GRANOLA BAR:** | | |
| *Nature Valley:* | | |
| Regular: | | |
| Almond or cinnamon | 1 piece | 120 |
| Coconut | 1 piece | 130 |
| Chewy: | | |
| Apple | 1 piece | 130 |
| Peanut butter | 1 piece | 140 |
| *New Trail:* | | |
| Chocolate chip or peanut butter | 1.3-oz. piece | 200 |
| Cocoa creme | 1.3-oz. piece | 90 |
| **\*GRANOLA BAR MIX,** chewy, | | |
| *Nature Valley, Bake-A-Bar* | 1 bar | 100 |
| **GRANOLA CEREAL:** | | |
| *Nature Valley:* | | |
| Cinnamon & raisin, fruit & nut or | | |
| toasted oat | ⅓ cup | 130 |
| Coconut & honey | ⅓ cup | 150 |
| *Sun Country:* | | |
| With almonds | 1 oz. | 130 |
| With raisins & dates | 1 oz. | 130 |
| **GRANOLA CLUSTERS,** | | |
| *Nature Valley:* | | |
| Almond | 1 piece | 140 |
| Caramel & raisin | 1 piece | 150 |
| **GRANOLA & FRUIT BAR,** | | |
| *Nature Valley* | 1 bar | 150 |
| **GRANOLA SNACK:** | | |
| *Nature Valley* | 1 pouch | 140 |
| *Kudos* (M&M/Mars): | | |
| Chocolate chip | 1¼-oz. piece | 180 |
| Peanut butter | 1.3-oz. piece | 190 |
| *Nature Valley* | 1 piece | 140 |
| **GRAPE:** | | |
| American, ripe (slipskin) | 3½″ × 3″ bunch | 43 |
| Canned, dietetic (Featherweight) | | |
| light, seedless, water pack | ½ cup | 60 |

| Food and Description | Measure or Quantity | Calories |
|---|---|---|
| **GRAPE DRINK:** | | |
| Canned: | | |
| *Bama* (Borden) | 8.45-fl.-oz. | 120 |
| *Capri Sun* | 6¾ fl. oz. | 104 |
| (Hi-C) | 6 fl. oz. | 89 |
| (Johanna Farms) *Ssips* | 8.45-fl.-oz. | 130 |
| (Lincoln) | 6 fl. oz. | 90 |
| (Welchade) | 6 fl. oz. | 90 |
| Chilled (Sunkist) | 8.45 fl. oz. | 140 |
| *Frozen (Welchade) | 6 fl. oz. | 90 |
| *Mix: | | |
| Regular (Hi-C) | 6 fl. oz. | 68 |
| Dietetic (Sunkist) | 8 fl. oz. | 6 |
| **GRAPEFRUIT:** | | |
| Pink & red: | | |
| Seeded type | ½ med. grapefruit | 46 |
| Seedless type | ½ med. grapefruit | 49 |
| White: | | |
| Seeded type | ½ med. grapefruit | 44 |
| Seedless type | ½ med. grapefruit | 46 |
| Canned, regular pack (Del Monte) in syrup | ½ cup | 74 |
| Canned, dietetic pack, solids & liq.: | | |
| (Del Monte) sections | ½ cup | 45 |
| (Diet Delight) sections | ½ cup | 45 |
| (Featherweight) sections, juice pack | ½ cup | 40 |
| (S&W) *Nutradiet* | ½ cup | 40 |
| **GRAPEFRUIT DRINK,** canned (Lincoln) | 6 fl. oz. | 104 |
| **GRAPEFRUIT JUICE:** | | |
| Fresh, pink, red or white | ½ cup | 46 |
| Canned, sweetened: | | |
| (Ardmore Farms) | 6 fl. oz. | 78 |
| (Del Monte) | 6 fl. oz. | 89 |
| (Texsun) | 6 fl. oz. | 77 |
| Canned, unsweetened: | | |
| (Del Monte) | 6 fl. oz. | 72 |
| (Ocean Spray) | 6 fl. oz. | 64 |
| (Texsun) | 6 fl. oz. | 77 |
| Chilled (Sunkist) | 6 fl. oz. | 72 |
| **GRAPEFRUIT JUICE COCKTAIL,** canned (Ocean Spray) pink | 6 fl. oz. | 84 |
| **GRAPEFRUIT-ORANGE JUICE COCKTAIL,** canned, Musselman's | 6 fl. oz. | 67 |
| **GRAPE JAM** (Smucker's) | 1 T. | 53 |
| **GRAPE JELLY:** | | |
| Sweetened: | | |
| *Bama* (Borden) | 1 T. | 45 |

| Food and Description | Measure or Quantity | Calories |
|---|---|---|
| (Smucker's) | 1 T. | 53 |
| (Welch's) | 1 T. | 52 |
| Dietetic: | | |
| (Diet Delight) | 1 T. | 12 |
| (Estee) | 1 T. | 6 |
| (Welch's) | 1 T. | 30 |
| **GRAPE JUICE:** | | |
| Canned, unsweetened: | | |
| (Ardmore Farms) | 6 fl. oz. | 99 |
| (Johanna Farms) *Tree Ripe* | 8.45-fl.-oz. | 164 |
| (Seneca Foods) | 6 fl. oz. | 118 |
| (Tree Top) sparkling | 6 fl. oz. | 120 |
| (Welch's) regular or red | 6 fl. oz. | 120 |
| *Frozen: | | |
| (Minute Maid) | 6 fl. oz. | 99 |
| (Welch's) | 6 fl. oz. | 100 |
| ***GRAPE JUICE DRINK,** frozen | | |
| (Sunkist) | 6 fl. oz. | 69 |
| *GRAPE NUTS,* cereal (Post): | | |
| Regular | ¼ cup (1 oz.) | 110 |
| Flakes | ⅞ cup (1 oz.) | 100 |
| **GRAVY,** canned: | | |
| Au jus (Franco-American) | 2-oz. serving | 5 |
| Beef (Franco-American) | 2-oz. serving | 25 |
| Brown: | | |
| (Estee) dietetic | ¼ cup | 14 |
| (Franco-American) with onion | 2-oz. serving | 25 |
| (Howard Johnson's) | ½ cup | 51 |
| (La Choy) | 2 oz. | 140 |
| *Ready Gravy* | ¼ cup | 44 |
| Chicken (Franco-American): | | |
| Regular | 2-oz. serving | 50 |
| Giblet | 2-oz. serving | 26 |
| Chicken & herb | ¼ cup | 20 |
| Mushroom (Franco-American) | 2-oz. serving | 25 |
| Pork (Franco-American) | 2-oz. serving | 40 |
| Turkey: | | |
| (Franco-American) | 2-oz. serving | 30 |
| (Howard Johnson's) giblet | ½ cup | 55 |
| *GRAVYMASTER* | 1 tsp. | 11 |
| **GRAVY MIX:** | | |
| Regular: | | |
| Au jus: | | |
| *(Durkee) | ½ cup | 15 |
| *(French's) *Gravy Makins* | ½ cup | 20 |
| Brown: | | |
| *(Durkee) regular | ½ cup | 29 |
| *(French's) *Gravy Makins* | ½ cup | 40 |
| *(Lawry's) | ½ cup | 47 |

| Food and Description | Measure or Quantity | Calories |
|---|---|---|
| *(Pillsbury) | ½ cup | 30 |
| *(Spatini) | 1 oz. | 8 |
| Chicken: | | |
| *(Durkee) regular | ½ cup | 43 |
| *(French's) *Gravy Makins* | ½ cup | 50 |
| *(Pillsbury) | ½ cup | 50 |
| Home style: | | |
| *(Durkee) | ½ cup | 35 |
| *(French's) *Gravy Makins* | ½ cup | 40 |
| *(Pillsbury) | ½ cup | 30 |
| Meatloaf (Durkee) *Roasting Bag* | 1.5-oz. pkg. | 129 |
| Mushroom: | | |
| *(Durkee) | ½ cup | 30 |
| *(French's) *Gravy Makins* | ½ cup | 40 |
| Onion: | | |
| *(Durkee) | ½ cup | 42 |
| *(French's) *Gravy Makins* | ½ cup | 50 |
| *(McCormick) | .85-oz. pkg. | 72 |
| Pork: | | |
| *(Durkee) | ½ cup | 35 |
| *(French's) *Gravy Makins* | ½ cup | 40 |
| *Swiss Steak (Durkee) | ½ cup | 23 |
| Turkey: | | |
| *(Durkee) | ½ cup | 47 |
| *(French's) *Gravy Makins* | ½ cup | 50 |
| *Dietetic (ESTEE): | | |
| Brown | ½ cup | 28 |
| Chicken | ½ cup | 40 |
| **GRAVY WITH MEAT OR TURKEY,** | | |
| Frozen: | | |
| (Banquet): | | |
| *Entree for One,* & sliced beef | 4 oz. | 90 |
| *Family Entree,* & sliced turkey | 32-oz. pkg. | 640 |
| (Morton) Light, sliced turkey | 8 oz. | 270 |
| (Swanson) sliced beef | 8-oz. entree | 200 |
| ***GREAT BEGINNINGS*** | | |
| (Hormel): | | |
| With chunky beef | 5 oz. | 136 |
| With chunky chicken | 5 oz. | 147 |
| With chunky turkey | 5 oz. | 138 |
| **GREENS, MIXED,** canned: | | |
| (Allens) | ½ cup | 25 |
| (Sunshine) solids & liq. | ½ cup | 20 |
| **GRENADINE** (Garnier) no alcohol | 1 fl. oz. | 103 |
| **GUACAMOLE SEASONING MIX** | | |
| (Lawry's) | .7-oz. pkg. | 60 |
| **GUAVA** | 1 guava | 48 |
| **GUAVA NECTAR** (Libby's) | 6 fl. oz. | 70 |

# H

| Food and Description | Measure or Quantity | Calories |
|---|---|---|
| **HADDOCK:** | | |
| Fried, breaded | 4" × 3" × ½" fillet | 165 |
| Frozen: | | |
| (Gorton's) *Light Recipe,* fillet entree | 1 piece | 260 |
| (Mrs. Paul's) breaded & fried crispy, crunchy | 2-oz. fillet | 140 |
| (Van de Kamp's) batter dipped, french fried | 2-oz. piece | 120 |
| (Weight Watchers) with stuffing, 2-compartment | 7-oz. pkg. | 205 |
| Smoked | 4-oz. serving | 117 |
| **HALIBUT:** | | |
| Broiled | 4" × 3" × ½" steak | 214 |
| Frozen (Van de Kamp's) batter dipped, french fried | ½ of 8-oz. pkg. | 260 |
| **HAM:** | | |
| Canned: | | |
| (Hormel): | | |
| *Black Label* (3- or 5-lb. size) | 4 oz. | 140 |
| Chunk | 6¾-oz. serving | 310 |
| Patties | 1 patty | 180 |
| (Oscar Mayer) *Jubilee,* extra lean, cooked | 1-oz. serving | 31 |
| (Swift) *Premium* | 1¾-oz. slice | 111 |
| Deviled: | | |
| (Hormel) | 1 T. | 35 |
| (Libby's) | 1 T. | 43 |
| (Underwood) | 1 T. | 49 |
| Packaged: | | |
| (Carl Buddig) smoked | 1 oz. | 50 |
| (Eckrich): | | |
| Loaf | 1 oz. | 70 |
| Cooked or imported, Danish | 1.2-oz. slice | 30 |
| (Hormel): | | |
| Black, or red peppered or frozen | 1 slice | 25 |
| Chopped | 1 slice | 55 |

| Food and Description | Measure or Quantity | Calories |
|---|---|---|
| (Ohse): | | |
| Chopped | 1 oz. | 65 |
| Cooked | 1 oz. | 30 |
| Smoked, regular | 1 oz. | 45 |
| (Oscar Mayer): | | |
| Chopped | 1-oz. slice | 52 |
| Cooked, smoked | ¾-oz. slice | 22 |
| *Jubilee,* boneless: | | |
| Sliced | 8-oz. slice | 232 |
| Steak, 95% fat free | 2-oz. steak | 58 |
| **HAM & ASPARAGUS BAKE,** frozen (Stouffer's) | 9½-oz. meal | 510 |
| **HAM & CHEESE:** | | |
| (Eckrich) loaf | 1-oz. serving | 60 |
| (Hormel) loaf | 1-oz. serving | 65 |
| (Ohse) loaf | 1 oz. | 65 |
| **HAM DINNER,** frozen: | | |
| (Banquet) American Favorites | 10-oz. dinner | 532 |
| (Morton) | 10-oz. dinner | 286 |
| **HAM SALAD,** canned (Carnation) | ¼ of 7½-oz. can | 110 |
| **HAM SALAD SPREAD** (Oscar Mayer) | 1 oz. | 59 |
| **HAMBURGER** (See *McDONALD'S, BURGER KING, DAIRY QUEEN, WHITE CASTLE,* etc.) | | |
| **HAMBURGER MIX:** | | |
| *\*Hamburger Helper* (General Mills): | | |
| Beef noodle or hamburger hash | ⅕ of pkg. | 320 |
| Cheeseburger macaroni or hamburger pizza dish | ⅕ of pkg. | 360 |
| Chili, with beans | ¼ of pkg. | 350 |
| Hamburger stew | ⅕ of pkg. | 300 |
| Lasagna | ⅕ of pkg. | 340 |
| Sloppy Joe bake | ⅕ of pkg. | 340 |
| Tamalebake | ⅕ of pkg. | 380 |
| *Make a Better Burger* (Lipton) mildly seasoned or onion | ⅕ pkg. | 30 |
| **HAMBURGER SEASONING MIX:** | | |
| *\*(Durkee) | 1 cup | 663 |
| (French's) | 1-oz. pkg. | 100 |
| **HARDEE'S:** | | |
| Apple turnover | 3.2-oz. piece | 270 |
| *Big Cookie* | 1.7-oz. piece | 260 |
| *Big Country Breakfast:* | | |
| Bacon | 7.65-oz. meal | 660 |
| Country ham | 8.96-oz. meal | 670 |
| Ham | 8.85-oz. meal | 620 |
| Sausage | 9.7-oz. meal | 850 |

| Food and Description | Measure or Quantity | Calories |
|---|---|---|
| Biscuit: | | |
|   Bacon | 3.3-oz. serving | 360 |
|   Bacon & egg | 4.4-oz. serving | 410 |
|   Bacon, egg & cheese | 4.8-oz. serving | 460 |
|   Chicken | 5.1-oz. serving | 430 |
|   Country ham: | | |
|     Plain | 3.8-oz. serving | 350 |
|     & egg | 4.9-oz. serving | 400 |
|     'n gravy | 7.8-oz. serving | 440 |
|   Ham: | | |
|     Plain | 3.7-oz. serving | 320 |
|     With egg | 4.9-oz. serving | 370 |
|     With egg & cheese | 5.3-oz. serving | 420 |
|   Rise 'N Shine: | | |
|     Plain | 2.9-oz. serving | 320 |
|     Canadian bacon | 5.7-oz. serving | 470 |
|   Sausage: | | |
|     Plain | 4.2-oz. serving | 440 |
|     With egg | 5.3-oz. serving | 490 |
|   Steak: | | |
|     Plain | 5.2-oz. serving | 500 |
|     With egg | 6.3-oz. serving | 550 |
| Cheeseburger: | | |
|   Plain | 4.3-oz. serving | 320 |
|   Bacon | 7.7-oz. serving | 610 |
|   Quarter-pound | 6.4-oz. serving | 500 |
| Chicken fillet sandwich | 6.1-oz. sandwich | 370 |
| Chicken, grilled, sandwich | 6.8-oz. sandwich | 310 |
| Chicken Stix: | | |
|   6-piece | 3½-oz. serving | 210 |
|   9-piece | 5.3-oz. serving | 310 |
| Cool Twist: | | |
|   Cone: | | |
|     Chocolate: | 4.2-oz. serving | 200 |
|     Vanilla | 4.2-oz. serving | 190 |
|     Vanilla/chocolate | 4.2-oz. serving | 190 |
|   Sundae: | | |
|     Caramel | 6-oz. serving | 330 |
|     Hot fudge | 5.9-oz. serving | 320 |
|     Strawberry | 5.9-oz. serving | 260 |
| Fisherman's Fillet, sandwich | 7.3-oz. sandwich | 500 |
| Hamburger: | | |
|   Plain | 3.9-oz. serving | 270 |
|   Big Deluxe | 7.6-oz. serving | 500 |
|   Mushroom 'N Swiss | 6.6-oz. serving | 490 |
| Hot dog, all beef | 4.2-oz. serving | 300 |
| Hot ham 'n cheese | 4.2-oz. sandwich | 330 |
| Margarine/butter blend | .2-oz. serving | 35 |

| Food and Description | Measure or Quantity | Calories |
|---|---|---|
| Pancakes, three: | | |
|   Plain | 4.8-oz. serving | 280 |
|   With sausage pattie | 6.2-oz. serving | 430 |
|   With bacon strips | 5.3-oz. serving | 350 |
| Potato: | | |
|   French fries: | | |
|     Regular | 2½-oz. order | 230 |
|     Large | 4-oz. order | 360 |
|     *Hash Rounds* | 2.8-oz. serving | 230 |
| Roast beef: | | |
|   Regular | 4-oz. serving | 260 |
|   *Big Roast Beef* | 4.7-oz. serving | 300 |
| Salads: | | |
|   Chef | 10.4-oz. serving | 240 |
|   Chicken & pasta | 14.6-oz. serving | 230 |
|   Garden | 8.5-oz. serving | 210 |
|   Side | 3.9-oz. serving | 20 |
| Shake: | | |
|   Chocolate | 12 fl. oz. | 460 |
|   Strawberry | 12 fl. oz. | 440 |
|   Vanilla | 12 fl. oz. | 400 |
| Syrup | 1½-oz. serving | 120 |
| Turkey club sandwich | 7.3-oz. serving | 390 |
| **HAWAIIAN PUNCH:** | | |
| Canned regular: | | |
|   Cherry or grape | 6 fl. oz. | 90 |
|   Orange | 6 fl. oz. | 100 |
| Canned, dietetic, punch | 6 fl. oz. | 30 |
| **HEADCHEESE** (Oscar Mayer) | 1-oz. serving | 55 |
| **HERRING,** canned (Vita): | | |
|   Cocktail, drained | 8-oz. jar | 342 |
|   In cream sauce | 8-oz. jar | 397 |
|   *Tastee Bits,* drained | 8-oz. jar | 361 |
| **HERRING, SMOKED,** kippered | 4-oz. serving | 239 |
| **HICKORY NUT,** shelled | 1 oz. | 191 |
| ***HO-HO*** (Hostess) | 1-oz. piece | 120 |
| **HOMINY,** canned (Allens) | | |
| golden, solids & liq. | ½ cup | 80 |
| **HOMINY GRITS:** | | |
| Dry: | | |
|   (Albers) | 1½ oz. | 150 |
|   (Aunt Jemima) | 3 T. | 102 |
|   (Quaker): | | |
|     Regular | 3 T. | 101 |
|     Instant: | | |
|       Regular | .8-oz. packet | 79 |
|       With imitation bacon or ham | 1-oz. packet | 101 |
| Cooked | 1 cup | 125 |
| **HONEY,** strained | 1 T. | 61 |

| Food and Description | Measure or Quantity | Calories |
|---|---|---|
| **HONEYCOMB,** cereal (Post) regular | 1⅓ cups | 112 |
| **HONEYDEW** | 2″ × 7″ wedge | 31 |
| **HONEY SMACKS,** cereal (Kellogg's) | ¾ cup | 110 |
| **HORSERADISH:** | | |
|   Raw, pared | 1 oz. | 25 |
|   Prepared (Gold's) | 1 tsp. | 4 |
| **HOSTESS O'S** (Hostess) | 2¾-oz. piece | 277 |

# I

| Food and Description | Measure or Quantity | Calories |
|---|---|---|
| **ICE CREAM** (Listed by type, such as sandwich, or *Whammy,* or by flavor—see also FROZEN DESSERT): | | |
| Almond (Good Humor) supreme | 4 fl. oz. | 350 |
| Almond amaretto (Baskin-Robbins) | 4 fl. oz. | 280 |
| Bar: | | |
| (Good Humor): | | |
| Chip candy crunch | 3-fl.-oz. bar | 255 |
| Chocolate Eclair | 3-fl.-oz. bar | 187 |
| Halo bar | 2½-fl.-oz. bar | 230 |
| Shark bar | 3-fl.-oz. bar | 68 |
| Strawberry shortcake | 3-fl.-oz. bar | 176 |
| Toasted almond | 3-fl.-oz. bar | 212 |
| Vanilla, chocolate coated | 3-fl.-oz. bar | 198 |
| (Häagen-Dazs): | | |
| Chocolate with dark chocolate coating | 1 bar | 360 |
| Vanilla with milk chocolate coating | 1 bar | 320 |
| Blueberry & cream (Häagen-Dazs) | 4 fl. oz. | 190 |
| *Bon Bon* (Carnation) vanilla | 1 piece | 33 |
| Butter Almond (Breyers) | ½ cup | 170 |
| Butter pecan: | | |
| (Breyer's) | ¼ pt. | 180 |
| (Häagen-Dazs) | 4 fl. oz. | 290 |
| (Lady Borden) | ½ cup | 180 |
| Cappuccino, (Baskin-Robbins) chip | 4 fl. oz. | 310 |
| Chocolate: | | |
| (Baskin-Robbins): | | |
| Regular | 4 fl. oz. | 264 |
| Mousse Royale | 4 fl. oz. | 293 |
| (Borden) old fashioned recipe | ½ cup | 130 |
| (Breyers) | ½ cup | 160 |
| (Good Humor) bulk | 4 fl. oz. | 130 |
| (Häagen-Dazs) mint | 4 fl. oz. | 290 |
| (Howard Johnson's) | ½ cup | 221 |
| Chocolate raspberry truffle (Baskin-Robbins) | 4 fl. oz. | 310 |
| Chocolate swirl (Borden) | ½ cup | 130 |

| Food and Description | Measure or Quantity | Calories |
|---|---|---|
| Coffee: | | |
| (Breyers) | ½ cup | 140 |
| (Häagen-Dazs) | 4 fl. oz. | 270 |
| Cookies & cream: | | |
| (Breyer's) | ½ cup | 170 |
| (Sealtest) | ½ cup | 150 |
| Cookie sandwich (Good Humor) | 2.7-fl.-oz. piece | 290 |
| *Eskimo Pie*, vanilla with chocolate coating | 3-fl.-oz. bar | 180 |
| *Eskimo, Thin Mint*, with chocolate coating | 2-fl.-oz. bar | 140 |
| *Fat Frog* (Good Humor) | 3-fl.-oz. pop | 154 |
| Fudge cake (Good Humor) | 6.3 fl. oz. | 214 |
| Fudge royal (Sealtest) | ½ cup | 140 |
| Grand marnier (Baskin-Robbins) | 4 fl. oz. | 240 |
| Honey (Häagen-Dazs) | 4 fl. oz. | 250 |
| *Jamocha* (Baskin-Robbins) | 1 scoop (2½ fl. oz.) | 146 |
| Jamocha almond fudge (Baskin-Robbins) | 4 fl. oz. | 270 |
| Jumbo Jet Star (Good Humor) | 4.5 fl. oz. | 84 |
| King cone (Good Humor) boysenberry | 5 fl.oz. | 340 |
| Key lime & cream (Häagen-Dazs) | 4 fl. oz. | 200 |
| Macadamia nut (Häagen-Dazs) | 4 fl. oz. | 280 |
| Maple walnut (Häagen-Dazs) | 4 fl. oz. | 310 |
| Milky pop (Good Humor) | 1.5-fl.-oz. piece | 46 |
| Mocha double nut (Häagen-Dazs) | 4 fl. oz. | 290 |
| Orange & cream (Häagen-Dazs) | 4 fl. oz. | 200 |
| *Oreo*, Cookies 'n Cream: | | |
| Bulk | 3 fl. oz. | 140 |
| Sandwich | 1 piece | 240 |
| Peach (Häagen-Dazs) | 4 fl. oz. | 212 |
| Pralines 'N Cream (Baskin-Robbins) | 1 scoop (2½ fl. oz.) | 177 |
| Rocky Road (Baskin-Robbins) | 4 fl. oz. | 300 |
| Rum raisin (Häagen-Dazs) | 4 fl. oz. | 250 |
| Sandwich (Good Humor) vanilla | 2½-oz. piece | 161 |
| Strawberry: | | |
| (Baskin-Robbins) wild, light | 4 fl. oz. | 90 |
| (Borden) | ½ cup | 130 |
| (Breyers) | ½ cup | 130 |
| (Häagen-Dazs) | 4 fl. oz. | 250 |
| (Howard Johnson's) | ½ cup | 187 |
| Strawberry & cream: | | |
| (Borden) old fashioned recipe | ½ cup | 130 |
| (Good Humor) | 4 fl. oz. | 94 |
| Supreme (Good Humor) milk | 4 fl. oz. | 278 |
| Vanilla: | | |
| (Baskin-Robbins) regular | 4 fl. oz. | 235 |
| (Borden) | ½ cup | 130 |

| Food and Description | Measure or Quantity | Calories |
|---|---|---|
| (Eagle Brand) | ½ cup | 150 |
| (Häagen-Dazs) | 4 fl. oz. | 260 |
| (Howard Johnson's) | ½ cup | 210 |
| (Sealtest) | ½ cup | 140 |
| Vanilla-chocolate cup | | |
| (Good Humor) | 6 fl. oz. | 201 |
| Vanilla cup (Good Humor) | 3 fl. oz. | 98 |
| Vanilla sandwich (Good Humor) | 3 fl. oz. | 191 |
| Vanilla swiss almond | | |
| (Häagen-Dazs) | 4 fl. oz. | 290 |
| *Whammy* (Good Humor) | | |
| assorted | 1.6-oz. piece | 95 |
| **ICE CREAM CONE,** cone only: | | |
| (Baskin-Robbins): | | |
| Sugar | 1 cone | 60 |
| Waffle | 1 cone | 140 |
| (Comet) sugar | 1 cone | 40 |
| **ICE CREAM CUP,** cup only | | |
| (Comet) regular | 1 cup | 20 |
| ***ICE CREAM MIX** (Salada) | | |
| any flavor | 1 cup | 310 |
| **ICE MILK:** | | |
| Hardened | ¼ pt. | 100 |
| Soft-serve | ¼ pt. | 133 |
| (Borden): | | |
| Chocolate | ½ cup | 100 |
| Vanilla | ½ cup | 90 |
| (Light 'n Lively) coffee | ½ cup | 100 |
| (Meadow Gold) vanilla, 4% fat | ¼ pt. | 95 |
| **ITALIAN DINNER,** frozen | | |
| (Banquet) | 12-oz. dinner | 597 |

# J

| Food and Description | Measure or Quantity | Calories |
|---|---|---|
| **JACK IN THE BOX RESTAURANT:** | | |
| Beef fajita pita sandwich | 6.2-oz. serving | 333 |
| Breadstick, sesame | .6-oz. piece | 70 |
| *Breakfast Jack* | 4.4-oz. serving | 307 |
| Burger: | | |
| Regular | 3.6-oz. serving | 267 |
| Cheeseburger: | | |
| Regular | 4-oz. serving | 315 |
| Bacon | 8.1-oz. serving | 705 |
| Double | 5¼-oz. serving | 467 |
| Ultimate | 9.9-oz. serving | 942 |
| *Jumbo Jack:* | | |
| Regular | 7.8-oz. serving | 584 |
| With cheese | 8.5-oz. serving | 677 |
| Swiss & bacon | 6.6-oz. serving | 678 |
| Cheesecake | 3.5-oz. serving | 309 |
| Chicken fajita pita sandwich | 6.7-oz. sandwich | 292 |
| Chicken fillet sandwich, grilled | 7.2-oz. sandwich | 408 |
| Chicken strips | 1 piece | 87 |
| Chicken supreme sandwich | 8.1-oz. serving | 575 |
| Coffee, black | 8 fl. oz. | 2 |
| Egg, scrambled, platter | 8.8-oz. serving | 662 |
| Egg roll | 1 piece | 135 |
| Fish supreme sandwich | 8-oz. sandwich | 554 |
| French fries: | | |
| Regular | 2.4-oz. order | 221 |
| Large | 3.8-oz. order | 353 |
| Jumbo | 4.8-oz. order | 442 |
| Jelly, grape | .5-oz. serving | 38 |
| Ketchup | 1 serving | 10 |
| Mayonnaise | 1 serving | 152 |
| Milk, low fat | 8 fl. oz. | 122 |
| Milk shake, any flavor | 10 oz. | 320 |
| Mustard | 1 serving | 8 |
| Onion rings | 3.8-oz. serving | 382 |
| Orange juice | 6.5-oz. serving | 80 |
| Pancake platter | 8.1-oz. serving | 612 |
| Salad: | | |
| Chef | 13-oz. salad | 295 |

| Food and Description | Measure or Quantity | Calories |
|---|---|---|
| Mexican chicken | 15.2-oz. salad | 443 |
| Side | 3.9-oz. salad | 51 |
| Taco | 14.8-oz. salad | 641 |
| Salad dressing: | | |
| Regular: | | |
| Blue cheese | 1.2-oz. serving | 131 |
| Buttermilk | 1.2-oz. serving | 181 |
| Thousand Island | 1.2-oz. serving | 156 |
| Dietetic or low calorie, French | 1.2-oz. serving | 80 |
| Sauce: | | |
| *A-1* | 1.8-oz. serving | 35 |
| BBQ | .9-oz. serving | 44 |
| Guacamole | .9-oz. serving | 55 |
| Mayo-mustard | .8-oz. serving | 124 |
| Mayo-onion | .8-oz. serving | 143 |
| Salsa | .9-oz. serving | 8 |
| Seafood cocktail | 1-oz. serving | 32 |
| Sweet & sour | 1-oz. serving | 40 |
| Sausage crescent | 5.5-oz. serving | 585 |
| Shrimp | 1 piece (.3 oz.) | 27 |
| Soft drink: | | |
| Sweetened: | | |
| *Coca-Cola Classic* | 12 fl. oz. | 144 |
| *Dr. Pepper* | 12 fl. oz. | 144 |
| Root beer, *Ramblin'* | 12 fl. oz. | 176 |
| *Sprite* | 12 fl. oz. | 144 |
| Diet, *Coca-Cola* | 12 fl. oz. | Tr. |
| Supreme crescent | 5.1-oz. serving | 547 |
| Syrup, pancake | 1.5-oz. serving | 121 |
| Taco: | | |
| Regular | 2.9-oz. serving | 191 |
| Super | 4.8-oz. serving | 288 |
| Taquito | 1-oz. piece | 73 |
| Tea, iced, plain | 12 fl. oz. | 3 |
| Tortilla chips | 1 oz. | 139 |
| Turnover, hot apple | 4.2-oz. piece | 410 |
| ***JELL-O FRUIT BAR*** | 1 bar | 45 |
| ***JELL-O FRUIT & CREAM BAR*** | 1 bar | 72 |
| ***JELL-O GELATIN POPS*** | 1 pop | 35 |
| ***JELL-O PUDDING POPS:*** | | |
| Chocolate, chocolate with chocolate chips & vanilla with chocolate chips | 1 bar | 80 |
| Chocolate covered chocolate & vanilla | 1 bar | 130 |
| **JELLY,** sweetened (See also individual flavors) | | |
| (Crosse & Blackwell) all flavors | 1 T. | 51 |

| Food and Description | Measure or Quantity | Calories |
|---|---|---|
| **JERUSALEM ARTICHOKE,** pared | 4 oz. | 75 |
| **JOHANNISBERG RIESLING WINE** | | |
| (Louis M. Martini) | 3 fl. oz. | 68 |
| ***JUST RIGHT,*** cereal | | |
| (Kellogg's) fruit, nut & flake | ¾ cup | 140 |

# K

| Food and Description | Measure or Quantity | Calories |
|---|---|---|
| **KABOOM**, cereal (General Mills) | 1 cup | 110 |
| **KALE:** | | |
| Boiled, leaves only | 4 oz. | 110 |
| Canned (Allen's) chopped, solids & liq. | ½ cup | 25 |
| Frozen: | | |
| (Birds Eye) chopped | ⅓ pkg. | 32 |
| (Frosty Acres) | 3.3 oz. | 25 |
| (McKenzie) chopped | 3⅓ oz. | 30 |
| (Southland) chopped | ⅕ of 16-oz. pkg. | 25 |
| **KARO SYRUP** (See SYRUP) | | |
| **KEFIR** (Alta-Dena Dairy): | | |
| Plain | 1 cup | 180 |
| Flavored | 1 cup | 190 |
| **KENTUCKY FRIED CHICKEN:** | | |
| Biscuit, buttermilk | 2.3-oz. serving | 232 |
| Chicken: | | |
| Original recipe: | | |
| Breast: | | |
| Center | 1 piece | 283 |
| Side | 1 piece | 267 |
| Drumstick | 1 piece | 146 |
| Thigh | 1 piece | 294 |
| Wing | 1 piece | 178 |
| Extra crispy: | | |
| Breast: | | |
| Center | 1 piece | 353 |
| Side | 1 piece | 354 |
| Drumstick | 1 piece | 173 |
| Thigh | 1 piece | 371 |
| Wing | 1 piece | 218 |
| *Chicken Littles* | 1.7-oz. sandwich | 169 |
| Chicken nugget | 1 piece | 46 |
| Cole slaw | 3.2-oz. serving | 119 |
| Corn on the cob | 5-oz. serving | 176 |
| Potatoes: | | |
| French fries | 2.7-oz. regular order | 244 |
| Mashed, & gravy | 3½-oz. serving | 71 |

| Food and Description | Measure or Quantity | Calories |
|---|---|---|
| Salad: | | |
|   Chicken topper | 8.4-oz. serving | 158 |
|   Garden: | | |
|     Large | 6.5-oz. serving | 76 |
|     Mini | 4.6-oz. serving | 28 |
| Salad dressing: | | |
|   Regular: | | |
|     Blue cheese | 1 T. | 72 |
|     Buttermilk | 1 T. | 74 |
|     French | 1 T. | 54 |
|     Thousand Island | 1 T. | 57 |
|   Dietetic, vinergrette | 1 T. | 18 |
| Sauce: | | |
|   Barbecue | 1-oz. serving | 35 |
|   Honey | .5-oz. serving | 49 |
|   Mustard | 1-oz. serving | 36 |
|   Sweet & sour | 1-oz. serving | 58 |
| **KIDNEY:** | | |
|   Beef, braised | 4 oz. | 286 |
|   Calf, raw | 4 oz. | 128 |
|   Lamb, raw | 4 oz. | 119 |
| **KIELBASA** (see **SAUSAGE,** Polish-style) | | |
| **_KING VITAMAN,_** cereal (Quaker) | 1¼ cups | 113 |
| **KIPPER SNACKS** (King David Brand) Norwegian | 3¼-oz. can | 195 |
| **KIWI FRUIT** (Calavo) | 1 fruit (5 oz., edible portion) | 45 |
| **_KIX,_** cereal | 1½ cups | 110 |
| **KNOCKWURST**(Hebrew National) | 3 oz. | 263 |
| **_KOO KOOS_** (Dolly Madison) | 1.5-oz. piece | 190 |
| ***KOOL-AID** (General Foods): | | |
|   Unsweetened (sugar to be added) | 8 fl. oz. | 98 |
|   Pre-sweetened: | | |
|     Regular, sugar sweetened: | | |
|       Apple or sunshine punch | 8 fl. oz. | 96 |
|       Cherry or grape | 8 fl. oz. | 89 |
|       Tropical punch | 8 fl. oz. | 99 |
|     Dietetic, sugar-free: | | |
|       Cherry or grape | 8 fl. oz. | 2 |
|       Sunshine punch | 8 fl. oz. | 4 |
| **KUMQUAT,** flesh & skin | 5 oz. | 74 |

# L

| Food and Description | Measure or Quantity | Calories |
|---|---|---|
| **LAMB:** | | |
| Leg: | | |
| Roasted, lean & fat | 3 oz. | 237 |
| Roasted, lean only | 3 oz. | 158 |
| Loin, one 5-oz. chop (weighed with bone before cooking) will give you: | | |
| Lean & fat | 2.8 oz. | 280 |
| Lean only | 2.3 oz. | 122 |
| Rib, one 5-oz. chop (weighed with bone before cooking) will give you: | | |
| Lean & fat | 2.9 oz. | 334 |
| Lean only | 2 oz. | 118 |
| Shoulder: | | |
| Roasted, lean & fat | 3 oz. | 287 |
| Roasted, lean only | 3 oz. | 174 |
| **LASAGNA:** | | |
| Dry: | | |
| (Buitoni) precooked | 1 sheet | 48 |
| (Mueller's) | 1 oz. | 105 |
| Canned (Hormel) *Short Orders* | 7½-oz. can | 260 |
| Frozen: | | |
| (Armour) *Dinner Classics* | 10-oz. meal | 380 |
| (Buitoni): | | |
| Regular | 9-oz. serving | 342 |
| Al forno | 8-oz. serving | 327 |
| Meat sauce | 5-oz. serving | 212 |
| (Celentano): | | |
| Regular | ½ of 16-oz. pkg. | 320 |
| Primavera | 11-oz. pkg. | 300 |
| (Conagra) *Light & Elegant* | 11¼-oz. entree | 280 |
| (Le Menu) vegetable | 11-oz. dinner | 360 |
| (Stouffer's): | | |
| Regular, plain | 10½-oz. meal | 360 |
| *Lean Cuisine:* | | |
| With meat sauce | 10¼-oz. meal | 270 |
| Zucchini | 11-oz. meal | 260 |
| (Swanson): | | |
| *Hungry Man*, with meat | 18¾-oz. dinner | 730 |

| Food and Description | Measure or Quantity | Calories |
|---|---|---|
| Main Course, with meat | 13¼-oz. entree | 450 |
| (Weight Watcher's) regular | 12-oz. meal | 360 |
| **LATKES,** frozen (Empire Kosher): | | |
| Mini | 3-oz. serving | 190 |
| Triangles | 3-oz. serving | 140 |
| **LEEKS** | 4 oz. | 59 |
| **LEMON:** | | |
| Whole | 2⅛" lemon | 22 |
| Peeled | 2⅛" lemon | 20 |
| **LEMONADE:** | | |
| Canned: | | |
| (Ardmore Farms) | 6 fl. oz. | 89 |
| Capri Sun | 6¾ fl. oz. | 63 |
| Country Time | 6 fl. oz. | 69 |
| Chilled (Minute Maid) regular or pink | 6 fl. oz. | 79 |
| *Frozen: | | |
| Country Time, regular or pink | 6 fl. oz. | 68 |
| (Sunkist) | 6 fl. oz. | 92 |
| *Mix: | | |
| Regular: | | |
| Country Time, regular or pink | 6 fl. oz. | 68 |
| (Hi-C) | 6 fl. oz. | 76 |
| Kool-Aid, sweetened, regular or pink | 6 fl. oz. | 65 |
| (Wyler's) regular | 6 fl. oz. | 61 |
| Dietetic: | | |
| Crystal Light | 8 fl. oz. | 4 |
| Kool-Aid | 6 fl. oz. | 3 |
| (Sunkist) | 8 fl. oz. | 8 |
| **LEMONADE BAR** (Sunkist) | 3-fl.-oz. bar | 68 |
| **LEMON EXTRACT** (Virginia Dare) | 1 tsp. | 21 |
| **LEMON JUICE:** | | |
| Canned, *ReaLemon* | 1 fl. oz. | 6 |
| *Frozen (Sunkist) unsweetened | 1 fl. oz. | 7 |
| ***LEMON-LIMEADE DRINK,** | | |
| Crystal Light | 8 fl. oz. | 4 |
| **LEMON PEEL,** candied | 1 oz. | 90 |
| **LEMON & PEPPER SEASONING** | | |
| (Lawry's) | 1 tsp. | 6 |
| **LENTIL,** cooked, drained | ½ cup | 107 |
| **LETTUCE:** | | |
| Bibb or Boston | 4" head | 23 |
| Cos or Romaine, shredded or broken into pieces | ½ cup | 4 |
| Grand Rapids, Salad Bowl or Simpson | 2 large leaves | 9 |
| Iceberg, New York or Great Lakes | ¼ of 4¾" head | 15 |
| ***LIFE,** cereal (Quaker) regular or cinnamon | ⅔ cup | 105 |

| Food and Description | Measure or Quantity | Calories |
|---|---|---|
| **LIME,** peeled | 2″ dia. | 15 |
| ***LIMEADE,** frozen (Minute Maid) | 6 fl. oz. | 75 |
| **LIME JUICE,** *ReaLime* | 1 T. | 2 |
| **LINGUINI,** frozen (Stouffer's) | | |
| clam sauce | 10½ oz. | 285 |
| **LIVER:** | | |
| Beef: | | |
| Fried | 6½″ × 2⅜″ × ⅜″ slice | 195 |
| Cooked (Swift) | 3.2-oz. serving | 141 |
| Calf, fried | 6½″ × 2⅛″ × ⅜″ slice | 222 |
| Chicken, simmered | 2″ × 2″ × ⅝″ piece | 41 |
| **LIVERWURST SPREAD** (Hormel) | 1-oz. serving | 70 |
| **LOBSTER:** | | |
| Cooked, meat only | 1 cup | 138 |
| Canned, meat only | 4-oz. serving | 108 |
| Frozen, South African lobster tail | | |
| 3 in 8-oz. pkg. | 1 piece | 87 |
| 4 in 8-oz. pkg. | 1 piece | 65 |
| 5 in 8-oz. pkg. | 1 piece | 51 |
| **LOBSTER NEWBURG** | 1 cup | 485 |
| **LOBSTER PASTE,** canned | 1-oz. serving | 51 |
| **LOBSTER SALAD** | 4-oz. serving | 125 |
| **LONG ISLAND TEA COCKTAIL** | | |
| (Mr. Boston) 12½% alcohol | 3 fl. oz. | 93 |
| ***LONG JOHN SILVER'S:*** | | |
| Catfish: | | |
| Dinner | 13.2-oz. serving | 860 |
| Fillet | 2½-oz. piece | 180 |
| Catsup | .4-oz. packet | 15 |
| Chicken plank: | | |
| Dinner: | | |
| 3-piece | 13-oz. serving | 830 |
| 4-piece | 14.6-oz. serving | 940 |
| Single piece | 1.6-oz. piece | 110 |
| Children's meals: | | |
| Chicken planks | 7.1-oz. serving | 510 |
| Fish | 6½-oz. serving | 440 |
| Fish & chicken planks | 8.1-oz. serving | 550 |
| Chowder, clam, with cod | 7-oz. serving | 140 |
| Clam: | | |
| Breaded | 2.3-oz. serving | 240 |
| Dinner | 12.8-oz. serving | 980 |
| Cod, entree, broiled | 5.4-oz. serving | 160 |
| Cole slaw, drained on fork | 3.4-oz. serving | 140 |
| Corn on the cob, with whirl | 6.6-oz. ear | 270 |
| Cracker, *Club* | .2-oz. package | 35 |
| Fish, battered | 2.6-oz. piece | 150 |
| Fish dinner, 3-piece | 16.1-oz. serving | 960 |

| Food and Description | Measure or Quantity | Calories |
|---|---|---|
| Fish dinner, home-style: | | |
| 3-piece | 13.1-oz. serving | 880 |
| 4-piece | 14.8-oz. serving | 1,010 |
| 6-piece | 18.1-oz. serving | 1,260 |
| Fish & fries, entree: | | |
| 2-piece | 10-oz. serving | 660 |
| 3-piece | 12.6-oz. serving | 810 |
| Fish, homestyle | 1.6-oz. piece | 125 |
| Fish & more | 13.4-oz. entree | 800 |
| Fish sandwich, homestyle | 6.9-oz. serving | 510 |
| Fish sandwich platter, homestyle | 13.4-oz. serving | 870 |
| Flounder, broiled | 5.1-oz. piece | 180 |
| Gumbo, with cod & shrimp bobs | 7-oz. serving | 110 |
| Halibut steak, broiled | 4.1-oz. serving | 140 |
| Hushpuppie | .8-oz. piece | 70 |
| Pie: | | |
| Lemon meringue | 4.2-oz. slice | 260 |
| Pecan | 4.4-oz. slice | 530 |
| Potato: | | |
| Baked, without topping | 7.1-oz. serving | 150 |
| Fries | 3-oz. serving | 220 |
| Rice pilaf | 3-oz. serving | 150 |
| Roll, dinner, plain | .9-oz. piece | 70 |
| Salad: | | |
| Garden | 8.7-oz. serving | 170 |
| Ocean chef | 11.3-oz. serving | 250 |
| Seafood, entree | 11.9-oz. serving | 270 |
| Side | 4.3-oz. serving | 20 |
| Salad dressing: | | |
| Regular: | | |
| Bleu cheese | 1.5-oz packet | 120 |
| Ranch | 1.5-oz. packet | 140 |
| Sea salad | 1.6-oz. packet | 140 |
| Dietetic, Italian | 1.6-oz. packet | 18 |
| Salmon, broiled | 4.4-oz. piece | 180 |
| Sauce: | | |
| Honey mustard | 1.2-oz. packet | 60 |
| Seafood | 1.2-oz. packet | 45 |
| Sweet & sour | 1.2-oz. packet | 60 |
| Tartar | 1-oz. packet | 80 |
| Seafood platter | 14.1-oz. entree | 970 |
| Shrimp, battered | .5-oz. piece | 40 |
| Shrimp, breaded | 2.2-oz. serving | 190 |
| Shrimp dinner, battered: | | |
| 6-piece | 11.1-oz. serving | 740 |
| 9-piece | 12.6-oz. serving | 860 |
| Shrimp feast, breaded: | | |
| 13-piece | 12.6-oz. serving | 880 |
| 21-piece | 14.8-oz. serving | 1070 |

| Food and Description | Measure or Quantity | Calories |
|---|---|---|
| Shrimp, fish & chicken dinner | 13.4-oz. dinner | 840 |
| Shrimp & fish dinner | 12.3-oz. dinner | 770 |
| Vegetables, mixed | 4-oz. serving | 60 |
| Vinegar, malt | .4-oz. packet | 2 |
| **LOQUAT,** fresh, flesh only | 2 oz. | 27 |
| *LUCKY CHARMS,* cereal (General Mills) | 1 cup | 110 |
| **LUNCHEON MEAT** (See also individual listings such as BOLOGNA, HAM, etc.): | | |
| Banquet loaf (Eckrich) | ¾-oz. slice | 50 |
| Bar-B-Que loaf (Oscar Mayer) | 1-oz. slice | 46 |
| Beef, jellied loaf (Hormel) | 1.2-oz. slice | 45 |
| Gourmet loaf (Eckrich) | 1-oz. slice | 35 |
| Ham & cheese (See HAM & CHEESE) | | |
| Honey loaf: | | |
| (Eckrich) | 1-oz. slice | 40 |
| (Hormel) | 1 slice | 55 |
| (Oscar Mayer) | 1-oz. slice | 34 |
| Iowa brand (Hormel) | 1 slice | 45 |
| Liver cheese (Oscar Mayer) | 1.3-oz. slice | 114 |
| Liver loaf (Hormel) | 1 slice | 80 |
| Luncheon loaf (Ohse) | 1 oz. | 75 |
| Macaroni-cheese loaf (Eckrich) | 1-oz. slice | 68 |
| Meat loaf | 1-oz. serving | 57 |
| New England brand sliced sausage: | | |
| (Eckrich) | 1-oz. slice | 35 |
| (Oscar Mayer) 92% fat free | .8-oz. slice | 29 |
| Old fashioned loaf (Oscar Mayer) | 1-oz. slice | 62 |
| Olive loaf: | | |
| (Eckrich) | 1-oz. slice | 80 |
| (Hormel) | 1-oz. slice | 55 |
| (Oscar Mayer) | 1-oz. slice | 60 |
| Peppered loaf: | | |
| (Eckrich) | 1-oz. slice | 40 |
| (Hormel) Light & Lean | 1 slice | 50 |
| (Oscar Mayer) 93% fat free | 1-oz. slice | 39 |
| Pickle loaf: | | |
| (Eckrich) | 1-oz. slice | 80 |
| (Hormel) | 1 slice | 60 |
| (Ohse) | 1 oz. | 60 |
| Pickle & pimiento (Oscar Mayer) | 1-oz. slice | 62 |
| Spiced (Hormel) | 1 slice | 75 |

# M

| Food and Description | Measure or Quantity | Calories |
|---|---|---|
| **MACADAMIA NUT** | | |
| (Royal Hawaiian) | 1 oz. | 197 |
| **MACARONI:** | | |
| Dry: | | |
| Spinach (Creamette) ribbons | 1 oz. | 105 |
| Whole wheat (Pritikin) | 1 oz. | 110 |
| Cooked: | | |
| 8–10 minutes, firm | 1 cup | 192 |
| 14–20 minutes, tender | 1 cup | 155 |
| Canned (Franco-American) *PizzOs* | 7½-oz. can | 170 |
| Frozen: | | |
| (Morton) & beef | 10-oz. dinner | 245 |
| (Swanson) & beef | 12-oz. dinner | 360 |
| **MACARONI & CHEESE:** | | |
| Canned: | | |
| (Franco-American) regular or elbow | 7⅜-oz. serving | 170 |
| (Hormel) *Short Orders* | 7½-oz. can | 170 |
| Frozen: | | |
| (Banquet): | | |
| Casserole | 8-oz. pkg. | 344 |
| Dinner | 9-oz. dinner | 334 |
| (Birds Eye) For One | 5¾-oz. pkg. | 304 |
| (Celentano) baked | ½ of 12-oz. pkg. | 290 |
| (Conagra) *Light & Elegant* | 9-oz. entree | 300 |
| (Morton) | 20-oz. casserole | 648 |
| (Stouffer's) | 6-oz. serving | 250 |
| (Swanson) | 12¼-oz. dinner | 380 |
| Mix: | | |
| *(Kraft): | | |
| Regular, plain | ¼ box | 190 |
| *Velveeta*, shells | ¼ box | 270 |
| *(Prince) | ¾ cup | 268 |
| **MACARONI & CHEESE LOAF,** packaged (Ohse) | 1 oz. | 60 |
| **MACARONI & CHEESE PIE,** frozen (Swanson) | 7-oz. pie | 210 |
| ***MACARONI SALAD MIX** (Betty Crocker) creamy | ⅙ of pkg. | 200 |

| Food and Description | Measure or Quantity | Calories |
|---|---|---|
| **MACKEREL,** Atlantic, broiled with fat | 8½" × 2½" × ½" fillet | 248 |
| *MAGIC SHELL* (Smucker's) | 1 T. | 95 |
| **MAI TAI COCKTAIL MIX** (Holland House): | | |
| Instant | .56-oz. envelope | 64 |
| Liquid | 1 oz. | 32 |
| **MALTED MILK MIX** (Carnation): | | |
| Chocolate | 3 heaping tsps. | 85 |
| Natural | 3 heaping tsps. | 88 |
| **MALT LIQUOR,** *Colt 45* | 12 fl. oz. | 156 |
| *MALT-O-MEAL,* cereal | 1 T. | 33 |
| **MANDARIN ORANGE** (See TANGERINE) | | |
| **MANGO,** fresh | 1 med. mango | 88 |
| **MANGO NECTAR** (Libby's) | 6 fl. oz. | 60 |
| **MANHATTAN COCKTAIL** (Mr. Boston) 20% alcohol | 3 fl. oz. | 123 |
| **MANHATTAN COCKTAIL MIX** (Holland House) liquid | 1 oz. | 28 |
| **MANICOTTI,** frozen: | | |
| (Buitoni): | | |
| Cheese | 5.5 oz. | 310 |
| Florentine | 2 manicotti | 284 |
| (Celentano): | | |
| Without sauce | 1 manicotti | 85 |
| With sauce | 1 manicotti | 150 |
| *MANWICH* (Hunt's) | 5.8-oz. serving | 310 |
| **MAPLE SYRUP** (See SYRUP, Maple) | | |
| **MARGARINE:** | | |
| Regular: | 1 pat (1" × 1.3" × 1", 5 grams) | 36 |
| (Mazola) | 1 T. | 104 |
| (Parkay) regular, soft or squeeze | 1 T. | 101 |
| Imitation or dietetic: | | |
| (Parkay) | 1 T. | 55 |
| (Weight Watchers) | 1 T. | 50 |
| Whipped (Blue Bonnet; Miracle; Parkay) | 1 T. | 67 |
| **MARGARITA COCKTAIL** (Mr. Boston): | | |
| Regular | 3 fl. oz. | 105 |
| Strawberry | 3 fl. oz. | 138 |
| **MARINADE MIX:** | | |
| Chicken (Adolph's) | 1-oz. packet | 64 |
| Meat: | | |
| (French's) | 1-oz. pkg. | 80 |
| (Kikkoman) | 1-oz. pkg. | 64 |

| Food and Description | Measure or Quantity | Calories |
|---|---|---|
| **MARJORAM** (French's) | 1 tsp. | 4 |
| **MARMALADE:** | | |
| Sweetened: | | |
| (Home Brands) | 1 T. | 52 |
| (Keiller) | 1 T. | 60 |
| (Smucker's) | 1 T. | 53 |
| Dietetic: | | |
| (Estee; Louis Sherry) | 1 T. | 6 |
| (Featherweight) | 1 T. | 16 |
| (S&W) *Nutradiet*, red label | 1 T. | 12 |
| *MARSHMALLOW FLUFF* | 1 heaping tsp. | 59 |
| *MARSHMALLOW KRISPIES,* cereal | | |
| (Kellogg's) | 1¼ cups | 140 |
| **MARTINI COCKTAIL** (Mr. Boston): | | |
| Gin, extra dry, 20% alcohol | 3 fl. oz. | 99 |
| Vodka, 20% alcohol | 3 fl. oz. | 102 |
| *MASA HARINA* (Quaker) | ⅓ cup | 137 |
| *MASA TRIGO* (Quaker) | ⅓ cup | 149 |
| **MATZO** (Manischewitz): | | |
| Regular: | | |
| Plain | 1-oz piece | 110 |
| Egg | 1 cracker | 108 |
| Miniature | 1 cracker | 9 |
| Tam Tam | 1 cracker | 15 |
| Wheat | 1 cracker | 9 |
| Dietetic: | | |
| Tam Tam, unsalted | 1 cracker | 14 |
| Thins | .8 oz. piece | 91 |
| **MATZO FARFEL** | | |
| (Manischewitz) | ½ cup | 143 |
| **MAYONNAISE:** | | |
| Real: | | |
| (Bennett's) | 1 T. | 110 |
| *Blue Plate* (Luzianne) | 1 T. | 100 |
| *Hellmann's* (Best Foods) | 1 T. | 103 |
| (Kraft) | 1 T. | 100 |
| (Rokeach) | 1 T. | 100 |
| Imitation or dietetic: | | |
| *Blue Plate* (Luzianne) | 1 T. | 50 |
| (Estee) | 1 T. | 45 |
| (Diet Delight) *Mayo-Lite* | 1 T. | 24 |
| (Featherweight) *Soyamaise* | 1 T. | 100 |
| *Hellmann's* (Best Foods) | 1 T. | 50 |
| (Kraft) light | 1 T. | 45 |
| (Pritikin) *Sweetlite* | 1 T. | 50 |
| (Weight Watchers) | 1 T. | 40 |
| *MAYPO,* cereal: | | |
| 30-second | ¼ cup | 89 |
| Vermont style | ¼ cup | 121 |

| Food and Description | Measure or Quantity | Calories |
|---|---|---|
| **McDONALD'S:** | | |
| Big Mac | 1 hamburger | 560 |
| Biscuit: | | |
|   With bacon, egg & cheese | 1 order | 440 |
|   With sausage | 1 order | 440 |
|   With sausage & egg | 1 order | 520 |
| Cheeseburger | 1 cheeseburger | 310 |
| *Chicken McNuggets* | 1 serving | 290 |
| *Chicken McNuggets Sauce:* | | |
|   Barbecue | 1.1-oz. serving | 50 |
|   Honey | .5-oz. serving | 45 |
|   Hot mustard | 1.1-oz. serving | 70 |
| Cookies: | | |
|   Chocolate chip | 1 package | 330 |
|   *McDonaldland* | 1 package | 290 |
| Danish: | | |
|   Apple or cheese, iced | 1 piece | 390 |
|   Cinnamon raisin | 1 piece | 440 |
| *Egg McMuffin* | 1 serving | 290 |
| Egg, scrambled | 1 serving | 140 |
| English muffin, with butter | 1 muffin | 170 |
| *Filet-O-Fish* | 1 sandwich | 440 |
| Grapefruit juice | 6 fl. oz. | 80 |
| Hamburger | 1 hamburger | 260 |
| Hot cakes with butter & syrup | 1 serving | 410 |
| *McD.L.T.* | 1 sandwich | 580 |
| Milk, 2% butterfat | 8 fl. oz. | 120 |
| Orange juice | 6 fl. oz. | 80 |
| Pie, apple | 1 pie | 260 |
|   Cherry | 1 pie | 260 |
| Potato: | | |
|   Fried | 1 small order | 220 |
|   Hash browns | 1 order | 130 |
| *Quarter Pounder:* | | |
|   Regular | 1 hamburger | 410 |
|   With cheese | 1 hamburger | 520 |
| Salad: | | |
|   Chef's salad | 1 serving | 230 |
|   Garden salad | 1 serving | 110 |
|   Side salad | 1 serving | 60 |
| Salad Bar: | | |
|   Bacon bits | 1 packet | 15 |
|   Chow mein noodles | 1 packet | 45 |
|   Croutons | 1 packet | 50 |
| Salad Dressings: | | |
|   Blue cheese | 1 packet (.5 oz.) | 70 |
|   French | 1 packet (.5 oz.) | 58 |
|   Thousand Island | 1 packet (.5 oz.) | 78 |
|   Lo-cal vinaigrette | 1 packet (.5 oz.) | 15 |

| Food and Description | Measure or Quantity | Calories |
|---|---|---|
| *Sausage McMuffin:* | | |
| Plain | 1 sandwich | 370 |
| With egg | 1 sandwich | 440 |
| Sausage, pork | 1 serving | 180 |
| Shake: | | |
| Chocolate | 1 serving | 390 |
| Strawberry | 1 serving | 350 |
| Vanilla | 1 serving | 380 |
| Soft drinks: | | |
| Sweetened: | | |
| *Coca-Cola,* classic | 12 fl. oz. | 144 |
| Orange drink | 12 fl. oz. | 133 |
| *Sprite* | 12 fl. oz. | 144 |
| Dietetic, *Coke* | 12 fl. oz. | 1 |
| Sundae: | | |
| Caramel | 1 serving | 340 |
| Hot fudge | 1 serving | 310 |
| Strawberry | 1 serving | 280 |
| Vanilla soft-serve, with cone | 1 serving | 140 |
| **MEATBALL DINNER or ENTREE,** frozen: | | |
| (Green Giant) sweet & sour | 9.9-oz. entree | 370 |
| (Swanson) | 8¼-oz. entree | 290 |
| **\*MEATBALL SEASONING MIX** | | |
| (Durkee) Italian style | 1 cup | 619 |
| **MEATBALL STEW:** | | |
| Canned *Dinty Moore* (Hormel) | 7½-oz. serving | 245 |
| Frozen (Stouffer's) *Lean Cuisine* | 10-oz. serving | 240 |
| **MEATBALLS, SWEDISH,** frozen: | | |
| (Armour) *Dinner Classics* | 12½-oz. meal | 480 |
| (Stouffer's) with noodles | 11-oz. pkg. | 480 |
| **MEAT LOAF DINNER,** frozen: | | |
| (Banquet): | | |
| Dinner | 11-oz. dinner | 395 |
| Entree for One | 5-oz. | 240 |
| (Morton) | 10-oz. dinner | 306 |
| (Swanson) with tomato sauce | 9-oz. entree | 310 |
| **MEAT LOAF SEASONING MIX:** | | |
| \*(Bell's) | 4½ oz. | 300 |
| (Contadina) | 3¾-oz. pkg. | 360 |
| **MEAT, POTTED:** | | |
| (Hormel) | 1 T. | 30 |
| (Libby's) | 1-oz. serving | 55 |
| **MEAT TENDERIZER:** | | |
| Regular (Adolph's; McCormick) | 1 tsp. | 2 |
| Seasoned (McCormick) | 1 tsp. | 5 |
| **MELBA TOAST,** salted | | |
| (Old London): | | |
| Garlic, onion or white rounds | 1 piece | 10 |

| Food and Description | Measure or Quantity | Calories |
|---|---|---|
| Pumpernickel, rye, wheat or white | 1 piece | 17 |
| **MELON BALL,** in syrup, frozen | ½ cup | 72 |
| **MENUDO,** canned (Hormel) | | |
| *Casa Grande* | 7½-oz. can | 90 |
| **MERLOT WINE** (Louis M. Martini) | | |
| 12½% alcohol | 3 fl. oz. | 63 |
| **MEXICALI DOGS,** frozen (Hormel) | 5-oz. serving | 400 |
| **MEXICAN DINNER,** frozen: | | |
| (Morton) | 11-oz. dinner | 300 |
| (Patio) fiesta | 12¼-oz. meal | 461 |
| (Swanson) | 16-oz. dinner | 580 |
| (Van de Kamp's) combination | 11½-oz. dinner | 420 |
| *MILK BREAK BARS* (Pillsbury): | | |
| Chocolate or chocolate mint | 1 bar | 230 |
| Natural | 1 bar | 220 |
| **MILK, CONDENSED,** *Eagle Brand* | | |
| (Borden) | 1 T. | 64 |
| *MILK, DRY,** non-fat, instant (Alba; | | |
| Carnation; Pet; *Sanalac*) | 1 cup | 80 |
| **MILK, EVAPORATED:** | | |
| Regular: | | |
| (Carnation) | 1 fl. oz. | 42 |
| (Pet) | 1 fl. oz. | 43 |
| Filled (Pet) | ½ cup | 150 |
| Low fat (Carnation) | 1 fl. oz. | 27 |
| Skimmed, (Carnation; *Pet 99*) | 1 fl. oz. | 25 |
| **MILK, FRESH:** | | |
| Buttermilk (Friendship) | 8 fl. oz. | 120 |
| Chocolate: | | |
| (Borden) *Dutch Brand* | 8 fl. oz. | 180 |
| (Hershey's) | 8 fl. oz. | 190 |
| (Johanna): | | |
| Regular | 8 fl. oz. | 200 |
| Lowfat | 8 fl. oz. | 150 |
| (Nestlé) *Quik* | 8 fl. oz. | 220 |
| Low fat: | | |
| (Borden): | | |
| 1% milkfat | 8 fl. oz. | 100 |
| 2% milkfat, *Hi-Protein Brand* | 8 fl. oz. | 140 |
| (Johanna): | | |
| Regular: | | |
| 1% lowfat | 8 fl. oz. | 100 |
| 2% lowfat, regular | 8 fl. oz. | 120 |
| Buttermilk | 8 fl. oz. | 120 |
| Skim (Borden) regular | 8 fl. oz. | 90 |
| Whole: | | |
| (Borden) regular or high calcium | 8 fl. oz. | 150 |
| (Johanna) | 8 fl. oz. | 150 |
| **MILK, GOAT,** whole | 1 cup | 163 |

| Food and Description | Measure or Quantity | Calories |
|---|---|---|
| **MILK, HUMAN** | 1 cup | 163 |
| *MILK MAKERS* (Swiss Miss): | | |
| Chocolate, malted or strawberry | 1 envelope or 1 tsp. | 18 |
| *Chocolate, malted or strawberry | 8 fl. oz. | 100 |
| *MILNOT,* dairy vegetable blend | 1 fl. oz. | 38 |
| **MINERAL WATER** (La Croix) | Any quantity | 0 |
| *MINI-WHEATS,* cereal (Kellogg's) | | |
| frosted | 1 biscuit | 28 |
| **MINT LEAVES** | ½ oz. | 4 |
| **MOLASSES:** | | |
| Barbados | 1 T. | 51 |
| Blackstrap | 1 T. | 40 |
| Dark (Brer Rabbit) | 1 T. | 33 |
| Light | 1 T. | 48 |
| Medium | 1 T. | 44 |
| Unsulphured (Grandma's) | 1 T. | 60 |
| **MORTADELLA** sausage | 1 oz. | 89 |
| *MOST,* cereal (Kellogg's) | ½ cup | 100 |
| **MOUSSE:** | | |
| Canned, dietetic (Featherweight) | | |
| chocolate | ½ cup | 100 |
| *Mix, dietetic (Pritikin): | | |
| Chocolate | ½ cup | 80 |
| Lemon or strawberry | ½ cup | 70 |
| *MÜESLIX,* cereal | | |
| (Kellogg's): | | |
| Bran | ½ cup | 130 |
| Five grain | ½ cup | 150 |
| **MUFFIN:** | | |
| Apple (Pepperidge Farm) with spice | 1 muffin | 170 |
| Blueberry: | | |
| (Morton) rounds | 1.5-oz. muffin | 110 |
| (Pepperidge Farm) | 1.9-oz. muffin | 180 |
| Bran (Pepperidge Farm) | 1 muffin | 180 |
| Carrot walnut (Pepperidge Farm) | 1 muffin | 170 |
| Chocolate chip (Pepperidge Farm) | 1 muffin | 170 |
| Corn: | | |
| (Morton) | 1.7-oz. muffin | 130 |
| (Pepperidge Farm) | 1.9-oz. muffin | 180 |
| English: | | |
| *Millbrook:* | | |
| Regular | 2-oz. muffin | 130 |
| Wholewheat | 2-oz. muffin | 120 |
| (Pepperidge Farm): | | |
| Plain | 2-oz. muffin | 140 |
| Cinnamon, raisin | 2-oz. muffin | 150 |
| (Pritikin) raisin | 2.3-oz. muffin | 150 |
| *Roman Meal* | 2.3-oz. muffin | 150 |
| (Thomas'): | | |

| Food and Description | Measure or Quantity | Calories |
|---|---|---|
| Regular or frozen or sourdough | 2-oz. muffin | 133 |
| Raisin | 2.2-oz. muffin | 153 |
| (Wonder) | 2-oz. muffin | 130 |
| Plain | 1.4-oz. muffin | 118 |
| Sourdough (Wonder) | 2-oz. muffin | 130 |
| **MUFFIN MIX:** | | |
| *Apple cinnamon (Betty Crocker) | 1/12 of pkg. | 120 |
| Blueberry: | | |
| *(Betty Crocker) wild | 1 muffin | 120 |
| (Duncan Hines) | 1/12 pkg. | 99 |
| Bran: | | |
| (Duncan Hines) | 1/12 pkg. | 97 |
| (Elam's) natural | 1 T. | 23 |
| *Cherry (Betty Crocker) | 1/12 pkg. | 120 |
| *Chocolate chip (Betty Crocker) | 1/12 of pkg. | 150 |
| *Corn, (Dromedary) | 1 muffin | 120 |
| **MULLIGAN STEW,** canned, | | |
| *Dinty Moore, Short Orders* (Hormel) | 7½-oz. can | 230 |
| **MUSCATEL WINE** (Gallo) | | |
| 14% alcohol | 3 fl. oz. | 86 |
| **MUSHROOM:** | | |
| Raw, whole | ½ lb. | 62 |
| Raw, trimmed, sliced | ½ cup | 10 |
| Canned (Green Giant) solids & liq., whole or sliced: | | |
| Regular | 2 oz. serving | 12 |
| B & B | ¼ cup serving | 12 |
| Frozen (Larsen) | 3½ oz. | 30 |
| **MUSHROOM, CHINESE,** dried | 1 oz. | 81 |
| **MUSSEL,** in shell | 1 lb. | 153 |
| **MUSTARD:** | | |
| Powder (French's) | 1 tsp. | 9 |
| Prepared: | | |
| Brown (French's; Gulden's) | 1 tsp. | 5 |
| Chinese (Chun King) | 1 tsp. | 5 |
| Dijon, *Grey Poupon* | 1 tsp. | 6 |
| Horseradish (Nalley's) | 1 tsp. | 5 |
| Yellow (Gulden's) | 1 tsp. | 5 |
| **MUSTARD GREENS:** | | |
| Canned (Allens) solids & liq. | ½ cup | 20 |
| Frozen: | | |
| (Birds Eye) | 1/3 pkg. | 25 |
| (Frosty Acres) | 3.3 oz. | 20 |
| (Southland) | 1/3 of 16-oz. pkg. | 20 |
| **MUSTARD SPINACH:** | | |
| Raw | 1 lb. | 100 |
| Boiled, drained, no added salt | 4-oz. serving | 18 |

# N

| Food and Description | Measure or Quantity | Calories |
|---|---|---|
| **NATHAN'S:** | | |
| French fries | Regular order | 550 |
| Hamburger | 1 sandwich | 360 |
| Hot dog & roll | 1 order | 290 |
| **NATURAL CEREAL:** | | |
| *Familia:* | | |
| Regular | ½ cup | 187 |
| Bran | ½ cup | 166 |
| No added sugar | ½ cup | 181 |
| *Heartland*: | | |
| Plain, coconut or raisin | ¼ cup | 130 |
| Trail mix | ¼ cup | 120 |
| (Quaker): | | |
| Hot, whole wheat | ⅓ cup | 106 |
| 100% | ¼ cup | 138 |
| 100% with raisins & dates | ¼ cup | 134 |
| **NATURE SNACKS** (Sun-Maid): | | |
| Carob Crunch | 1 oz. | 143 |
| Carob Peanut | 1¼ oz. | 190 |
| Carob Raisin or Yogurt Raisin | 1¼ oz. | 160 |
| Tahitian Treat or Yogurt Crunch | 1 oz. | 123 |
| **NECTARINE,** flesh only | 4 oz. | 73 |
| **NOODLE:** | | |
| Cooked, 1½″ strips | 1 cup | 200 |
| Dry (Pennsylvania Dutch Brand) broad | 1 oz. | 105 |
| **NOODLE, CHOW MEIN:** | | |
| (Chun King) | 1 oz. | 139 |
| (La Choy) | ½ cup (1 oz.) | 150 |
| **NOODLE MIX:** | | |
| *(Betty Crocker): | | |
| Fettucini Alfredo | ¼ pkg. | 220 |
| Stroganoff | ¼ pkg. | 240 |
| *(Lipton) & sauce: | | |
| Alfredo, carbonara | ¼ of pkg. | 140 |
| Butter | ¼ of pkg. | 152 |
| Cheese | ¼ of pkg. | 141 |
| Chicken | ¼ of pkg. | 131 |
| Parmesan | ¼ of pkg. | 143 |

| Food and Description | Measure or Quantity | Calories |
|---|---|---|
|    Stroganoff | ¼ of pkg. | 110 |
| *NOODLE, RAMEN, canned (La Choy): | | |
|   Beef or oriental | 1½ oz. | 190 |
|   Chicken | 1½ oz. | 187 |
| NOODLE, RICE (La Choy) | 1 oz. | 130 |
| NOODLE ROMANOFF, frozen (Stouffer's) | ⅓ pkg. | 170 |
| NOODLES & BEEF: | | |
|   Canned (Hormel) *Short Orders* | 7½-oz. can | 230 |
|   Frozen (Banquet) *Buffet Supper* | 2-lb. pkg. | 754 |
| NOODLES & CHICKEN: | | |
|   Canned (Hormel) *Dinty Moore, Short Orders* | 7½-oz. can | 210 |
|   Frozen (Swanson) | 10½-oz. dinner | 270 |
| NUT (See specific type: CASHEW, MACADAMIA, etc.) | | |
| *NUT & HONEY CRUNCH,* cereal (Kellogg's) | ⅔ cup | 110 |
| NUT, MIXED: | | |
|   Dry roasted: | | |
|     (Flavor House) | 1 oz. | 172 |
|     (Planters) salted | 1 oz. | 160 |
|   Honey roasted (Fisher) | 1 oz. | 150 |
|   Oil roasted (Planters) with or without peanuts | 1 oz. | 180 |
| NUTMEG (French's) | 1 tsp. | 11 |
| *NUTRIFIC,* cereal (Kellogg's) | 1 cup | 120 |
| *NUTRI-GRAIN,* cereal (Kellogg's): | | |
|   Corn | ½ cup | 100 |
|   Wheat | ⅔ cup | 100 |
|   Wheat & Raisin | ⅔ cup | 130 |
| *NUTRIMATO* (Mott's) | 6 fl. oz. | 70 |

# O

| Food and Description | Measure or Quantity | Calories |
| --- | --- | --- |
| **OAT FLAKES,** cereal (Post) | ⅔ cup | 107 |
| **OATMEAL:** | | |
| Dry: | | |
| Regular: | | |
| (Elam's) Scotch style | 1 oz. | 108 |
| (H-O) old fashioned | 1 T. | 15 |
| (3-Minute Brand) | ⅓ cup | 110 |
| Instant: | | |
| (H-O): | | |
| Regular, boxed | 1 T. | 15 |
| With bran & spice | 1½-oz. packet | 157 |
| With maple & brown sugar flavor | 1½-oz. packet | 160 |
| (Quaker): | | |
| Regular | 1-oz. packet | 105 |
| Apple & cinnamon | 1¼-oz. packet | 134 |
| Raisins & spice | 1½-oz. packet | 159 |
| (3-Minute Brand) | ½-oz. packet | 162 |
| *Total* (General Mills): | | |
| Regular | 1-oz. packet | 90 |
| Cinnamon raisin almond | 1½-oz. packet | 150 |
| Mixed nut | 1.3-oz. packet | 140 |
| Quick: | | |
| (Ralston Purina) | ⅓ cup | 110 |
| (3-Minute Brand) | ⅓ cup | 110 |
| *Total* (General Mills) | 1 oz. | 90 |
| Cooked, regular | 1 cup | 132 |
| **OIL, SALAD OR COOKING:** | | |
| (Bertoli) olive | 1 T. | 120 |
| (Calavo) avocado | 1 T. | 120 |
| *Crisco, Mazola* | 1 T. | 126 |
| *Mrs. Tucker's;* (Goya) | 1 T. | 130 |
| *Sunlite: Wesson* | 1 T. | 120 |
| **OKRA,** frozen: | | |
| (Birds Eye) whole, baby | ⅓ pkg. | 36 |
| (Frosty Acres): | | |
| Cut | 3.3 oz. | 25 |
| White | 3.3 oz. | 30 |
| (Larsen) cut | 3.3 oz. | 25 |

| Food and Description | Measure or Quantity | Calories |
|---|---|---|
| (Seabrook Farms) cut | ⅓ pkg. | 32 |
| (Southland) cut | ⅕ of 16-oz. pkg. | 30 |
| **OLD FASHIONED COCKTAIL** | | |
| (Hiram Walker) 62 proof | 3 fl. oz. | 165 |
| **OLIVE:** | | |
| Green | 4 med. or 3 extra large or 2 giant | 19 |
| Ripe (Lindsay) by size: | | |
| Colossal | .4-oz. olive | 9 |
| Extra large or large | .2-oz. olive | 6 |
| Medium or small | .1-oz. olive | 3 |
| Super colassal | .5-oz. olive | 11 |
| **OMELET,** frozen (Swanson) | | |
| *TV Brand,* Spanish style | 7¾-oz. entree | 240 |
| **ONION:** | | |
| Raw | 2½" onion | 38 |
| Boiled, pearl onion | ½ cup | 27 |
| Canned (Durkee) *O & C:* | | |
| Boiled | ¼ of 16-oz. jar. | 32 |
| Creamed | ¼ of 15½-oz. can | 554 |
| Dehydrated (Gilroy) flakes | 1 tsp. | 5 |
| Frozen: | | |
| (Birds Eye): | | |
| Creamed | ⅓ pkg. | 106 |
| Whole, small | ⅓ pkg. | 44 |
| (Frosty Acres) chopped | 1 oz. | 8 |
| (Green Giant) in cheese sauce | ½ cup | 90 |
| (Larsen): | | |
| Diced | 1 oz. | 8 |
| Whole | 3.3 oz. | 35 |
| (Mrs. Paul's) french-fried rings | ½ of 5-oz. pkg. | 167 |
| **ONION BOUILLON:** | | |
| (Herb-Ox) | 1 cube | 10 |
| *MBT* | 1 packet | 16 |
| (Wyler's) instant | 1 tsp. | 10 |
| **ONION, COCKTAIL** | | |
| (Vlasic) | 1 oz. | 4 |
| **ONION, GREEN** | 1 small onion | 4 |
| **ONION SALAD SEASONING** | | |
| (French's) instant | 1 T. | 15 |
| **ONION SALT** (French's) | 1 tsp. | 6 |
| **ONION SOUP** (See SOUP, Onion) | | |
| **ORANGE:** | | |
| Peeled | ½ cup | 62 |
| Sections | 4 oz. | 58 |
| **ORANGE-APRICOT JUICE COCKTAIL,** *Musselman's* | 8 fl. oz. | 100 |

| Food and Description | Measure or Quantity | Calories |
|---|---|---|
| **ORANGE DRINK:** | | |
| Canned: | | |
| *Bama* (Borden) | 8.45-fl.-oz. container | 120 |
| *Capri Sun* | 6¾-fl.-oz. can | 103 |
| (Hi-C) | 6 fl. oz. | 95 |
| (Lincoln) | 6 fl. oz. | 90 |
| *Ssips* (Johanna Farms) | 8.45-fl.-oz. container | 130 |
| *Mix: | | |
| Regular (Hi-C) | 8 fl. oz. | 91 |
| Dietetic: | | |
| *Crystal Light* | 6 fl. oz. | 4 |
| (Sunkist) | 6 fl. oz. | 6 |
| **ORANGE EXTRACT** (Durkee) imitation | 1 tsp. | 15 |
| **ORANGE FRUIT DRINK,** canned (Ardmore Farms) | 6 fl. oz. | 86 |
| **ORANGE-GRAPEFRUIT JUICE:** | | |
| Canned (Libby's) unsweetened | 6 fl. oz. | 80 |
| *Frozen (Minute Maid) unsweetened | 6 fl. oz. | 76 |
| **ORANGE JUICE:** | | |
| Canned: | | |
| (Borden) *Sippin' Pak* | 8.45-fl.-oz. container | 110 |
| (Del Monte) unsweetened | 6 fl. oz. | 80 |
| (Johanna Farms) | 6 fl. oz. | 84 |
| (Libby's) unsweetened | 6 fl. oz. | 90 |
| (Texsun) sweetened | 6 fl. oz. | 83 |
| Chilled (Sunkist) | 6 fl. oz. | 76 |
| *Frozen: | | |
| (Birds Eye) *Orange Plus* | 6 fl. oz. | 95 |
| *Bright & Early,* imitation | 6 fl. oz. | 90 |
| (Citrus Hill): | | |
| Regular | 6 fl. oz. | 90 |
| Lite | 6 fl. oz. | 60 |
| (Sunkist) | 6 fl. oz. | 84 |
| **ORANGE JUICE BAR** (Sunkist) | 3-fl. oz. bar | 72 |
| **ORANGE PEEL, CANDIED** | 1 oz. | 93 |
| **ORANGE-PINEAPPLE DRINK,** canned (Lincoln) | 6 fl. oz. | 90 |
| **ORANGE-PINEAPPLE JUICE,** canned (Texsun) | 8 fl. oz. | 89 |
| **ORCHARD BLEND JUICE,** canned (Welch's): | | |
| Apple-grape | 6 fl. oz. | 100 |
| Harvest | 6 fl. oz. | 90 |
| Vineyard | 6 fl. oz. | 120 |
| *OVALTINE,* chocolate | ¾ oz. | 78 |
| *OVEN FRY* (General Foods): | | |
| Crispy crumb for pork | 4.2-oz. envelope | 484 |
| Crispy crumb for chicken | 4.2-oz. envelope | 460 |

| Food and Description | Measure or Quantity | Calories |
|---|---|---|
| Homestyle flour recipe | 3.2-oz. envelope | 304 |
| **OYSTER:** | | |
| Raw: | | |
| Eastern | 19–31 small or 13–19 med. | 158 |
| Pacific & Western | 6–9 small or 4–6 med. | 218 |
| Canned (Bumble Bee) shelled, whole, solids & liq. | 1 cup | 218 |
| Fried | 4 oz. | 271 |
| **OYSTER STEW,** home recipe | ½ cup | 103 |

# P

| Food and Description | Measure or Quantity | Calories |
|---|---|---|
| **PAC-MAN,** cereal (General Mills) | 1 cup | 110 |
| ***PANCAKE BATTER,** frozen (Aunt Jemima): | | |
| Plain | 4″ pancake | 70 |
| Blueberry or buttermilk | 4″ pancake | 68 |
| **PANCAKE DINNER OR ENTREE,** frozen (Swanson): | | |
| & blueberry sauce | 7-oz. meal | 400 |
| & sausage | 6-oz. meal | 460 |
| **PANCAKE & SAUSAGE,** frozen (Swanson) | 6-oz. entree | 440 |
| ***PANCAKE & WAFFLE MIX:** | | |
| Plain: | | |
| (Aunt Jemima) Original | 4″ pancake | 73 |
| (Log Cabin) Complete | 4″ pancake | 58 |
| (Pillsbury) *Hungry Jack:* | | |
| Complete, bulk | 4″ pancake | 63 |
| *Extra Lights* | 4″ pancake | 70 |
| *Golden Blend*, complete | 4″ pancake | 80 |
| *Panshakes* | 4″ pancake | 83 |
| Blueberry (Pillsbury) *Hungry Jack* | 4″ pancake | 107 |
| Buckwheat (Aunt Jemima) | 4″ pancake | 67 |
| Buttermilk: | | |
| (Aunt Jemima) regular | 4″ pancake | 100 |
| (Betty Crocker) complete | 4″ pancake | 70 |
| (Pillsbury) *Hungry Jack,* complete | 4″ pancake | 63 |
| Whole wheat (Aunt Jemima) | 4″ pancake | 83 |
| Dietetic: | | |
| (Estee) | 3″ pancake | 33 |
| (Featherweight) | 4″ pancake | 43 |
| **PANCAKE & WAFFLE SYRUP** (See SYRUP, Pancake & Waffle) | | |
| **PAPAYA,** fresh: | | |
| Cubed | ½ cup | 36 |
| Juice | 4 oz. | 78 |
| **PAPRIKA** (French's) | 1 tsp. | 7 |
| **PARSLEY:** | | |
| Fresh, chopped | 1 T. | 2 |
| Dried (French's) | 1 tsp. | 4 |

| Food and Description | Measure or Quantity | Calories |
|---|---|---|
| **PASSION FRUIT,** giant, whole | 1 lb. | 53 |
| **PASTA DINNER OR ENTREE,** frozen: | | |
| (Birds Eye): | | |
| Continental | 5-oz. serving | 164 |
| Primavera, For One | 5-oz. serving | 204 |
| (Stouffer's): | | |
| Carbonara | 9¾-oz. meal | 620 |
| Mexicali | 10-oz. meal | 490 |
| Primavera | 10⅝-oz. meal | 270 |
| **PASTA SALAD:** | | |
| *Mix (Betty Crocker) *Suddenly Salads,* Italian | ⅙ of pkg. | 160 |
| Frozen (Birds Eye) classic, Italian style | ½ of 10-oz. pkg. | 170 |
| ***PASTA & SAUCE,** mix (Lipton): | | |
| Cheese supreme | ¼ of pkg. | 139 |
| Mushroom & chicken | ¼ of pkg. | 124 |
| Oriental, with fusilli | ¼ of pkg. | 130 |
| Tomato, herb | ¼ of pkg. | 130 |
| **PASTINAS,** egg | 1 oz. | 109 |
| **PASTRAMI** (Carl Buddig) | 1 oz. | 40 |
| **PASTRAMI,** packaged: | | |
| (Carl Buddig) smoked, sliced | 1 oz. | 40 |
| *Hebrew National,* first cut | 1 oz. | 44 |
| **PASTRY POCKETS** (Pillsbury) | 1 pocket | 230 |
| **PASTRY SHEET, PUFF,** frozen (Pepperidge Farm) | 1 sheet | 1150 |
| **PÂTE:** | | |
| De foie gras | 1 T. | 69 |
| Liver: | | |
| (Hormel) | 1 T. | 35 |
| (Sell's) | 1 T. | 93 |
| *PDQ:* | | |
| Chocolate | 1 T. | 66 |
| Strawberry | 1 T. | 60 |
| **PEA,** green: | | |
| Boiled | ½ cup | 58 |
| Canned, regular pack, solids & liq.: | | |
| (Comstock) | ½ cup | 70 |
| (Del Monte) seasoned or sweet, regular size | ½ cup | 60 |
| (Green Giant): | | |
| Early with onions, sweet or sweet with onions | ¼ of 17-oz. can | 60 |
| Sweet, mini | ¼ of 17-oz. can | 64 |
| (Larsen) *Fresh-Lite* | ½ cup | 50 |
| Canned, dietetic pack, solids & liq.: | | |
| (Del Monte) no salt added, sweet | ½ cup | 60 |

| Food and Description | Measure or Quantity | Calories |
|---|---|---|
| (Diet Delight) | ½ cup | 50 |
| (Featherweight) sweet | ½ cup | 70 |
| (Larsen) *Fresh-Lite*, low sodium | ½ cup | 50 |
| Frozen: | | |
| (Birds Eye): | | |
| Regular | ⅓ pkg. | 78 |
| In butter sauce | ⅓ pkg. | 85 |
| In cream sauce | ⅓ pkg. | 84 |
| (Frosty Acres): | | |
| Regular | 3.3 oz. | 80 |
| Tiny | 3.3 oz. | 60 |
| (Green Giant): | | |
| In cream sauce | ½ cup | 100 |
| Sweet, *Harvest Fresh* | ½ cup | 80 |
| **PEA & CARROT:** | | |
| Canned, regular pack, solids & liq.: | | - |
| (Comstock) | ½ cup | 60 |
| (Del Monte) | ½ cup | 50 |
| (Libby's) | ½ cup | 56 |
| (Veg-All) | ½ cup | 50 |
| Canned, dietetic pack, solids & liq.: | | |
| (Diet Delight) | ½ cup | 40 |
| (Larsen) *Fresh-Lite*, low sodium | ½ cup | 50 |
| (S&W) *Nutradiet* | ½ cup | 35 |
| Frozen: | | |
| (Birds Eye) | ⅓ pkg. | 61 |
| (Larsen) | 3.3 oz. | 60 |
| (McKenzie) | 3.3-oz. serving | 60 |
| **PEA, CROWDER,** frozen | | |
| (Southland) | ⅕ of 16-oz. pkg. | 130 |
| **PEA POD:** | | |
| Boiled, drained solids | 4 oz. | 49 |
| Frozen (La Choy) | 6-oz. pkg. | 70 |
| **PEACH:** | | |
| Fresh, with thin skin | 2″ dia. | 38 |
| Fresh slices | ½ cup | 32 |
| Canned, regular pack, solids & liq.: | | |
| (Del Monte) Cling: | | |
| Halves or slices | ½ cup | 80 |
| Spiced | 3½ oz. | 80 |
| (Hunt's) *Snack Pack* | 5-oz. container | 110 |
| (Libby's) heavy syrup: | | |
| Halves | ½ cup | 105 |
| Sliced | ½ cup | 102 |
| Canned, dietetic pack, solids & liq.: | | |
| (Del Monte) Lite, Cling | ½ cup | 50 |
| (Diet Delight) Cling: | | |
| Juice pack | ½ cup | 50 |
| Water Pack | ½ cup | 30 |

| Food and Description | Measure or Quantity | Calories |
|---|---|---|
| (Featherweight); | | |
| Cling or Freestone, juice | | |
| pack | ½ cup | 50 |
| Cling, water pack | ½ cup | 30 |
| (S&W) *Nutradiet*, Cling: | | |
| Juice pack | ½ cup | 60 |
| Water pack | ½ cup | 30 |
| Frozen (Birds Eye) | 5-oz. pkg. | 141 |
| **PEACH BUTTER** (Smucker's) | 1 T. | 45 |
| **PEACH DRINK,** canned (Hi-C): | | |
| Canned | 6 fl.oz. | 101 |
| *Mix | 6 fl. oz. | 72 |
| **PEACH LIQUEUR** (DeKuyper) | 1 fl. oz. | 82 |
| **PEACH NECTAR,** canned | | |
| (Ardmore Farms) | 6 fl. oz. | 90 |
| **PEACH PRESERVE OR JAM:** | | |
| Sweetened: | | |
| (Bama) | 1 T. | 45 |
| (Home Brands) | 1 T. | 50 |
| (Smucker's) | 1 T. | 53 |
| Dietetic (Dia-Mel) | 1 T. | 6 |
| **PEANUT:** | | |
| In shell (Planters) | 1 oz. | 160 |
| Dry roasted: | | |
| (Fisher) | 1 oz. | 163 |
| (Planters) | 1 oz. | 160 |
| (Tom's) | 1 oz. | 160 |
| Honey roasted: | | |
| (Eagle) | 1 oz. | 170 |
| (Fisher) | 1 oz. | 150 |
| Oil roasted (Planters) salted | 1 oz. | 170 |
| **PEANUT BUTTER:** | | |
| Regular: | | |
| (Adams) | 1 T. | 95 |
| (Bama) creamy or crunchy | 1 T. | 100 |
| (Elam's) natural | 1 T. | 109 |
| (Holsum) | 1 T. | 94 |
| (Home Brands) | 1 T. | 105 |
| (Laura Scudder's) | 1 T. | 95 |
| (Peter Pan) | 1 T. | 90 |
| (Skippy) creamy or super chunk | 1 T. | 95 |
| Dietetic: | | |
| (Adams) low sodium | 1 T. | 95 |
| (Home Brands): | | |
| Lightly salted or unsalted | 1 T. | 105 |
| No sugar added | 1 T. | 90 |
| (Peter Pan) creamy | 1 T. | 95 |
| (S&W) *Nutradiet,* low sodium | 1 T. | 93 |
| (Smucker's) low sodium | 1 T. | 100 |

| Food and Description | Measure or Quantity | Calories |
|---|---|---|
| **PEANUT BUTTER BAKING** | | |
| **CHIPS** (Reese's) | 3 T. (1 oz.) | 151 |
| ***PEANUT BUTTER BOPPERS*** | | |
| (General Mills): | | |
|     Cookie crunch or peanut crunch | 1 bar | 170 |
|     Fudge graham | 1 bar | 160 |
| **PEANUT BUTTER & JELLY** (Bama) | 1 T. | 75 |
| **PEANUT, SPANISH** | | |
| (Fisher): | | |
|     Raw | 1 oz. | 160 |
|     Roasted, oil | 1 oz. | 170 |
| (Planters): | | |
|     Raw | 1 oz. | 150 |
|     Roasted: | | |
|       Dry | 1 oz. | 160 |
|       Oil | 1 oz. | 170 |
| **PEAR:** | | |
|   Whole | 3″ × 2½″ pear | 101 |
|   Canned, regular pack, solids & liq.: | | |
|     (Del Monte) Bartlett | ½ cup | 80 |
|     (Libby's) | ½ cup | 102 |
|   Canned, dietetic pack, solids & liq.: | | |
|     (Del Monte) Lite | ½ cup | 50 |
|     (Featherweight) Bartlett: | | |
|       Juice pack | ½ cup | 60 |
|       Water pack | ½ cup | 40 |
|     (Libby's) water pack | ½ cup | 60 |
|   Dried (Sun-Maid) | ½ cup | 260 |
| **PEAR-APPLE JUICE** (Tree Top) | 6 fl. oz. | 90 |
| **PEAR-GRAPE JUICE** (Tree Top) | 6 fl. oz. | 100 |
| **PEAR NECTAR,** canned | | |
| (Ardmore Farms) | 6 fl. oz. | 96 |
| **PEAR-PASSION FRUIT NECTAR,** | | |
| canned (Libby's) | 6 fl. oz. | 60 |
| **PEAR, STRAINED** | | |
| (Larsen) | ½ cup | 65 |
| ***PEBBLES,*** cereal: | | |
|   Cocoa | ⅞ cup | 117 |
|   Fruity | ⅞ cup | 116 |
| **PECAN:** | | |
|   Halves | 6-7 pieces | 48 |
|   Roasted, dry: | | |
|     (Fisher) salted | 1 oz. | 220 |
|     (Planters) | 1 oz. | 190 |
| **PECTIN, FRUIT:** | | |
| *Certo* | 6-oz. pkg. | 19 |
| *Sure-Jell* | 1¾-oz. pkg. | 170 |
| **PEPPER:** | | |
|   Black (French's) | 1 tsp. | 9 |

| Food and Description | Measure or Quantity | Calories |
|---|---|---|
| Seasoned (French's) | 1 tsp. | 8 |
| **PEPPER & ONION,** frozen (Southland) | 2-oz. serving | 15 |
| **PEPPER, BANANA** (Vlasic) hot rings | 1 oz. | 4 |
| **PEPPER, CHERRY** (Vlasic) mild | 1 oz. | 8 |
| **PEPPER, CHILI,** canned: | | |
| (Del Monte): | | |
| Green, whole | ½ cup | 20 |
| Jalapeño or chili, whole | ½ cup | 30 |
| *Old El Paso,* green, chopped or whole | 1 oz. | 7 |
| (Ortega): | | |
| Diced, strips or whole | 1 oz. | 10 |
| Jalapeño, diced or whole | 1 oz. | 9 |
| (Vlasic) Jalapeño | 1 oz. | 8 |
| **PEPPERMINT EXTRACT** (Durkee) imitation | 1 tsp. | 15 |
| **PEPPERONCINI** (Vlasic) Greek, mild | 1 oz. | 4 |
| **PEPPERONI:** | | |
| (Eckrich) | 1-oz. serving | 135 |
| (Hormel) regular or Rosa Grande | 1-oz. serving | 140 |
| **PEPPER STEAK:** | | |
| *Canned (La Choy) | ¾ cup | 210 |
| Frozen: | | |
| (Armour) *Classic Lite,* beef | 10½-oz. dinner | 260 |
| (Blue Star) *Dining Lite,* with rice | 9½-oz. entree | 267 |
| (La Choy) Fresh & Lite, with rice & vegetables | 10-oz. meal | 280 |
| (Le Menu) | 11½-oz. dinner | 360 |
| (Stouffer's) | 10½-oz. serving | 330 |
| **PEPPER, STUFFED:** | | |
| Home recipe | 2¾″ × 2½″ pepper with 1⅛ cups stuffing | 314 |
| Frozen: | | |
| (Celentano) | 12½-oz. pkg. | 290 |
| (Stouffer's) green | 7¾-oz. serving | 200 |
| (Weight Watchers) with veal stuffing | 11¾-oz. meal | 270 |
| **PEPPER, SWEET:** | | |
| Raw: | | |
| Green: | | |
| Whole | 1 lb. | 82 |
| Without stem & seeds | 1 med. pepper (2.6 oz.) | 13 |
| Red: | | |
| Whole | 1 lb. | 112 |

122

| Food and Description | Measure or Quantity | Calories |
|---|---|---|
| Without stem & seeds | 1 med. pepper (2.2 oz.) | 19 |
| Boiled, green, without salt, drained | 1 med. pepper (2.6 oz.) | 13 |
| Frozen: | | |
| (Frosty Acres) diced: | | |
| Green | 1 oz. | 6 |
| Red & green | 1 oz. | 7 |
| (Larsen) green | 1 oz. | 6 |
| (McKenzie) | 1-oz. serving | 6 |
| (Southland) diced | 2-oz. serving | 10 |
| **PERCH, OCEAN:** | | |
| Atlantic, raw: | | |
| Whole | 1 lb. | 124 |
| Meat only | 4 oz. | 108 |
| Pacific, raw, whole | 1 lb. | 116 |
| Frozen: | | |
| (Banquet) | 8¾-oz. dinner | 434 |
| (Frionor) *Norway Gourmet* | 4 oz. fillet | 120 |
| (Mrs. Paul's) fillet, breaded & fried | 2-oz. piece | 145 |
| (Van de Kamp's) batter dipped, french fried | 2-oz. piece | 135 |
| **PERNOD** (Julius Wile) | 1 fl. oz. | 79 |
| **PERSIMMON:** | | |
| Japanese or Kaki, fresh: | | |
| With seeds | 4.4-oz. piece | 79 |
| Seedless | 4.4-oz. piece | 81 |
| Native, fresh, flesh only | 4-oz. serving | 144 |
| **PETITE SIRAH WINE** (Louis M. Martini): | | |
| Regular, 12% alcohol | 3 fl. oz. | 62 |
| White, 12.3% alcohol | 3 fl. oz. | 54 |
| **PHEASANT,** raw, meat only | 4-oz. serving | 184 |
| **PICKLE:** | | |
| Cucumber, fresh or bread & butter: | | |
| (Fannings) | 1.2-oz. serving | 17 |
| (Featherweight) low sodium | 1-oz. pickle | 12 |
| (Vlasic): | | |
| Chips | 1 oz. | 7 |
| Stix, sweet butter | 1 oz. | 5 |
| Dill: | | |
| (Featherweight) low sodium, whole | 1-oz. serving | 4 |
| (Smucker's): | | |
| Hamburger, sliced | 1 slice | Tr. |
| Polish, whole | 3½" pickle | 8 |
| (Vlasic): | | |
| Original | 1 oz. | 2 |

**123**

| Food and Description | Measure or Quantity | Calories |
|---|---|---|
| No garlic | 1 oz. | 4 |
| Hamburger (Vlasic) chips | 1-oz. serving | 2 |
| Hot & spicy (Vlasic) garden mix | 1 oz. | 4 |
| Kosher dill: | | |
| (Claussen) halves or whole | 2-oz. serving | 7 |
| (Featherweight) low sodium | 1-oz. serving | 4 |
| (Smucker's): | | |
| Baby | 2¾"-long pickle | 4 |
| Whole | 3½"-long pickle | 8 |
| (Vlasic) | 1 oz. | 4 |
| Sweet: | | |
| (Nalley's) *Nubbins* | 1-oz. serving | 28 |
| (Smucker's): | | |
| Gherkins | 2"-long pickle | 15 |
| Whole | 2½"-long pickle | 18 |
| (Vlasic) | 1 oz. | 30 |
| Sweet & sour (Claussen) slices | 1 slice | 3 |
| **PIE:** | | |
| Regular, non-frozen: | | |
| Apple: | | |
| Home recipe, two crust | ⅙ of 9" pie | 404 |
| (Dolly Madison) | 4½-oz. pie | 490 |
| (Hostess) | 4½-oz. pie | 390 |
| Banana, home recipe, cream or custard | ⅙ of 9" pie | 336 |
| Berry (Hostess) | 4½-oz. pie | 404 |
| Blackberry, home recipe, two-crust | ⅙ of 9" pie | 384 |
| Blueberry: | | |
| Home recipe, two-crust | ⅙ of 9" pie | 382 |
| (Dolly Madison) | 4½-oz. pie | 430 |
| (Hostess) | 4½-oz. pie | 394 |
| Boston cream, home recipe | 1/12 of 8" pie | 208 |
| Butterscotch, home recipe, one-crust | ⅙ of 9" pie | 406 |
| Cherry: | | |
| Home recipe, two-crust | ⅙ of 9" pie | 412 |
| (Dolly Madison) regular | 4½-oz. pie | 470 |
| (Hostess) | 4½-oz. pie | 390 |
| Chocolate (Dolly Madison): | | |
| Regular | 4½-oz. pie | 560 |
| Pudding | 4½-oz. pie | 500 |
| Chocolate chiffon, home recipe | ⅙ of 9" pie | 459 |
| Chocolate meringue, home recipe | ⅙ of 9" pie | 353 |
| Coconut custard, home recipe | ⅙ of 9" pie | 357 |
| Lemon (Hostess) | 4½-oz. pie | 400 |
| Lemon meringue, home recipe, one-crust | ⅙ of 9" pie | 357 |

| Food and Description | Measure or Quantity | Calories |
|---|---|---|
| Mince, home recipe, two-crust | ⅙ of 9″ pie | 428 |
| Peach (Dolly Madison) | 4½-oz. pie | 460 |
| Pumpkin, home recipe, one-crust | ⅙ of 9″ pie | 321 |
| Raisin, home recipe, two-crust | ⅙ of 9″ pie | 427 |
| Strawberry (Hostess) | 4½-oz. pie | 340 |
| Vanilla (Dolly Madison) pudding | 4½-oz. pie | 500 |
| Frozen: | | |
| Apple: | | |
| (Banquet) family size | ⅙ of 20-oz. pie | 253 |
| (Morton): | | |
| Regular | ⅙ of 24-oz. pie | 296 |
| *Great Little Desserts,* regular | 8-oz. pie | 590 |
| (Weight Watchers) | 3 oz. | 180 |
| Banana cream: | | |
| (Banquet) | ⅙ of 14-oz. pie | 172 |
| (Morton) regular | ⅙ of 16-oz. pie | 174 |
| Blackberry (Banquet) | ⅙ of 20-oz. pie | 268 |
| Blueberry: | | |
| (Banquet) | ⅙ of 20-oz. pie | 266 |
| (Morton) *Great Little Desserts* | 8-oz. pie | 580 |
| Cherry: | | |
| (Banquet) | ⅙ of 20-oz. pie | 252 |
| (Morton) regular | ⅙ of 24-oz. pie | 300 |
| (Weight Watchers) | 3 oz. | 200 |
| Chocolate (Morton) | ⅙ of 14-oz. pie | 180 |
| Chocolate cream: | | |
| (Banquet) | ⅙ of 14-oz. pie | 177 |
| (Morton) *Great Little Desserts* | 3½-oz. pie | 270 |
| Coconut cream (Banquet) | ⅙ of 14-oz. pie | 179 |
| Coconut custard (Morton) | | |
| *Great Little Desserts* | 6½-oz. pie | 370 |
| Lemon cream: | | |
| (Banquet) | ⅙ of 14-oz. pie | 168 |
| (Morton) *Great Little Desserts* | 3½-oz. pie | 250 |
| Mince: | | |
| (Banquet) | ⅙ of 20-oz. pie | 258 |
| (Morton) | ⅙ of 24-oz. pie | 310 |
| Peach (Sara Lee) | ⅙ of 31-oz. pie | 458 |
| Pumpkin: | | |
| (Banquet) | ⅙ of 20-oz. pie | 197 |
| (Morton) regular | ⅙ of 24-oz. pie | 230 |
| Strawberry cream (Banquet) | ⅙ of 14-oz. pie | 168 |
| **PIECRUST:** | | |
| Home recipe, 9″ pie | 1 crust | 900 |
| Frozen (Empire Kosher) | 7 oz. | 1001 |
| Refrigerated (Pillsbury) | 2 crusts | 1920 |
| ***PIECRUST MIX:** | | |
| (Betty Crocker): | | |
| Regular | ¹⁄₁₆ pkg. | 120 |

| Food and Description | Measure or Quantity | Calories |
|---|---|---|
| Stick | ⅛ stick | 120 |
| (Flako) | ⅙ of 9″ pie shell | 245 |
| (Pillsbury) mix or stick | ⅙ of 2-crust pie | 270 |
| **PIE FILLING** (See also **PUDDING OR PIE FILLING**): | | |
| Apple: | | |
| (Comstock) | ⅙ of 21-oz. can | 110 |
| (Thank You Brand) | 3½ oz. | 91 |
| (White House) | ½ cup | 163 |
| Apple rings or slices (See APPLE, canned) | | |
| Apricot (Comstock) | ⅙ of 21-oz. can | 110 |
| Banana cream (Comstock) | ⅙ of 21-oz. can | 110 |
| Blueberry (Comstock) | ⅙ of 21-oz. can | 120 |
| Cherry (Thank You Brand) regular | 3½ oz. | 99 |
| Coconut cream (Comstock) | ⅙ of 21-oz. can | 120 |
| Coconut custard, home recipe, made with egg yolk & milk | 5 oz. (inc. crust) | 288 |
| Lemon (Comstock) | ⅙ of 21-oz. can | 160 |
| Mincemeat (Comstock) | ½ of 21-oz. can | 170 |
| Peach (White House) | ½ cup | 158 |
| Pumpkin (Libby's) (See also PUMPKIN, canned) | 1 cup | 210 |
| Raisin (Comstock) | ⅙ of 21-oz. can | 140 |
| ***PIE MIX**: | | |
| Boston Cream (Betty Crocker) | ⅛ of pie | 270 |
| Chocolate (Royal) | ⅛ of pie | 260 |
| **PIEROGIES,** frozen: | | |
| (Empire Kosher): | | |
| Cheese | 1½ oz. | 110 |
| Onion | 1½ oz. | 90 |
| (Mrs. Paul's) potato & cheese | 1 piece | 90 |
| **PIGS FEET,** pickled | 4-oz. serving | 226 |
| **PIMIENTO,** canned: | | |
| (Dromedary) drained | 1-oz. serving | 10 |
| (Ortega) | ¼ cup | 6 |
| (Sunshine) diced or sliced | 1 T. | 4 |
| **PIÑA COLADA** (Mr. Boston) 12½% alcohol | 3 fl. oz. | 249 |
| ***PIÑA COLADA MIX** (Bar-Tender's) | 5 fl. oz. | 254 |
| **PINEAPPLE:** | | |
| Fresh, chunks | ½ cup | 52 |
| Canned, regular pack, solids & liq.: | | |
| (Del Monte) slices, syrup pack (Dole): | ½ cup | 90 |
| Juice pack, chunk, crushed or sliced | ½ cup | 70 |

126

| Food and Description | Measure or Quantity | Calories |
|---|---|---|
| Heavy syrup, chunk, crushed or sliced | ½ cup | 95 |
| Canned, unsweetened or dietetic, solids & liq.: | | |
| (Diet Delight) juice pack | ½ cup | 70 |
| (Libby's) Lite | ½ cup | 60 |
| (S&W) *Nutradiet* | 1 slice | 30 |
| **PINEAPPLE & GRAPEFRUIT JUICE DRINK,** canned: | | |
| (Del Monte) regular or pink | 6 fl. oz. | 90 |
| (Dole) pink | 6 fl. oz. | 101 |
| (Texsun) | 6 fl. oz. | 91 |
| **PINEAPPLE, CANDIED** | 1-oz. serving | 90 |
| **PINEAPPLE FLAVORING** (Durkee) imitation | 1 tsp. | 6 |
| **PINEAPPLE JUICE:** | | |
| Canned: | | |
| (Ardmore Farms) | 6 fl. oz. | 102 |
| (Dole) | 6 fl. oz. | 103 |
| (Texsun) | 6 fl. oz. | 97 |
| *Frozen (Minute Maid) | 6 fl. oz. | 92 |
| **PINEAPPLE-ORANGE DRINK,** canned (Hi-C) | 6 fl. oz. | 94 |
| **PINEAPPLE-ORANGE JUICE:** | | |
| Canned: | | |
| (Del Monte) | 6 fl. oz. | 90 |
| (Johanna Farms) *Tree Ripe* | 8.45-fl.-oz. container | 132 |
| *Frozen (Minute Maid) | 6 fl. oz. | 94 |
| **PINEAPPLE PRESERVE OR JAM,** sweetened (Home Brands) | 1 T. | 52 |
| **PINE NUT,** pignolias, shelled | 1 oz. | 156 |
| **PINOT CHARDONNAY WINE** (Paul Masson) 12% alcohol | 3 fl. oz. | 71 |
| **PISTACHIO NUT:** | | |
| In shell | ½ cup | 197 |
| Shelled | ¼ cup | 184 |
| (Fisher) shelled, roasted, salted | 1 oz. | 174 |
| **PIZZA PIE** (See also **SHAKEY'S**): | | |
| Regular, non-frozen: | | |
| Home recipe | ⅛ of 14" pie | 177 |
| (*Domino's*): | | |
| Beef, ground: | | |
| Plain: | | |
| 12" pizza (small) | 1 slice | 216 |
| 16" pizza (large) | 1 slice | 303 |
| With pepperoni: | | |
| 12" pizza (small) | 1 slice | 216 |
| 16" pizza (large) | 1 slice | 303 |
| Cheese: | | |

| Food and Description | Measure or Quantity | Calories |
|---|---|---|
| Plain: | | |
| 12″ pizza (small) | 1 slice | 157 |
| 16″ pizza (large) | 1 slice | 239 |
| Double cheese: | | |
| 12″ pizza (small) | 1 slice | 240 |
| 16″ pizza (large) | 1 slice | 350 |
| Double, with pepperoni | | |
| 12″ pizza (small) | 1 slice | 227 |
| 16″ pizza (large) | 1 slice | 389 |
| Mushroom & sausage: | | |
| 12″ pizza (small) | 1 slice | 183 |
| 16″ pizza (large) | 1 slice | 266 |
| Pepperoni: | | |
| Plain: | | |
| 12″ pizza (small) | 1 slice | 192 |
| 16″ pizza (large) | 1 slice | 278 |
| With mushrooms: | | |
| 12″ pizza (small) | 1 slice | 194 |
| 16″ pizza (large) | 1 slice | 280 |
| With sausage: | | |
| 12″ pizza (small) | 1 slice | 215 |
| 16″ pizza (large) | 1 slice | 303 |
| Sausage: | | |
| 12″ pizza (small) | 1 slice | 180 |
| 16″ pizza (large) | 1 slice | 264 |
| (Godfather's): | | |
| Cheese: | | |
| Original: | | |
| Mini | ¼ of pizza (2.8 oz.) | 190 |
| Small | ⅙ of pizza (3.6 oz.) | 240 |
| Medium | ⅛ of pizza (4½ oz.) | 270 |
| Large: | | |
| Regular | ¹⁄₁₀ of pizza (4.4 oz.) | 297 |
| Hot slice | ⅛ of pizza (5½ oz.) | 370 |
| Stuffed: | | |
| Small | ⅙ of pizza (4.4 oz.) | 310 |
| Medium | ⅛ of pizza (4.8 oz.) | 350 |
| Large | ¹⁄₁₀ of pizza (5.2 oz.) | 381 |
| Thin crust: | | |
| Small | ⅙ of pizza (2.6 oz.) | 180 |
| Medium | ⅛ of pizza (3 oz.) | 210 |
| Large | ¹⁄₁₀ of pizza (3.4 oz.) | 228 |
| Combo: | | |
| Original: | | |
| Mini | ¼ of pizza (3.8 oz.) | 240 |
| Small | ⅙ of pizza (5.6 oz.) | 360 |
| Medium | ⅛ of pizza (6.2 oz.) | 400 |
| Large: | | |
| Regular | ¹⁄₁₀ of pizza (6.8 oz.) | 437 |

| Food and Description | Measure or Quantity | Calories |
|---|---|---|
| Hot slice | ⅛ of pizza (8.5 oz.) | 550 |
| Stuffed: | | |
| Small | ⅙ of pizza (6.3 oz.) | 430 |
| Medium | ⅛ of pizza (7 oz.) | 480 |
| Large | ⅒ of pizza (7.6 oz.) | 521 |
| Thin crust: | | |
| Small | ⅙ of pizza (4.3 oz.) | 270 |
| Medium | ⅛ of pizza (4.9 oz.) | 310 |
| Large | ⅒ of pizza (5.4 oz.) | 336 |
| Frozen: | | |
| Bacon (Totino's) | ½ of 10-oz. pie | 370 |
| Bagel (Empire Kosher) | 2-oz. serving | 140 |
| Canadian style bacon (Celeste) | 8-oz. pie | 483 |
| Cheese: | | |
| (Celentano): | | |
| Mini slice | 1 slice | 157 |
| Thick crust | ⅓ of 13-oz. pie | 238 |
| (Empire Kosher): | | |
| Regular | ⅓ of 10-oz. pie | 195 |
| 3-pack | ⅑ of 27-oz. pie | 215 |
| (Stouffer's) French Bread: | | |
| Regular, double cheese | ½ of 11¾-oz. pkg. | 410 |
| Lean Cuisine, extra cheese | 5½-oz. serving | 350 |
| (Weight Watchers) | 6-oz. pie | 350 |
| Combination: | | |
| (Celeste) Chicago style | ¼ of 24-oz. pie | 360 |
| (La Pizzeria) | ½ of 13½-oz. pie | 420 |
| (Van de Kamp's) thick crust | ¼ of 24½-oz. pie | 310 |
| (Weight Watchers) | 7¼-oz. pie | 322 |
| Deluxe: | | |
| (Celeste) | ½ of 9-oz. pie | 281 |
| (Stouffer's) French Bread | ½ of 12⅜-oz. pkg. | 430 |
| English muffin (Empire Kosher) | 2-oz. serving | 140 |
| Hamburger (Stouffer's) French Bread | ½ of 12¼-oz. pkg. | 410 |
| Mushroom (Stouffer's) French Bread | ½ of 12-oz. pkg. | 340 |
| Pepperoni: | | |
| (Stouffer's) French Bread: | | |
| Regular | ½ of 11¼-oz. pkg. | 410 |
| Lean Cuisine | 5½-oz. serving | 340 |
| (Weight Watchers) | 6¼-oz. pie | 370 |
| Sausage: | | |
| (Celeste) | ½ of 8-oz. pie | 262 |
| (Stouffer's) French Bread | ½ of 12-oz. pkg. | 420 |
| (Weight Watchers) veal | 6¾-oz. pie | 350 |
| Sausage & mushroom: | | |
| (Celeste) | ¼ of 24-oz. pie | 365 |
| (Stouffer's) French Bread | ½ of 12½-oz. pkg. | 410 |

| Food and Description | Measure or Quantity | Calories |
|---|---|---|
| Sausage & pepperoni (Stouffer's) French Bread | ½ of 12½-oz. pkg. | 450 |
| Sicilian style (Celeste) deluxe | ¼ of 26-oz. pie | 408 |
| Supreme (Celeste) without meat | ½ of 8-oz. pie | 217 |
| Vegetable (Stouffer's) French Bread | ½ of 12¾-oz. pkg. | 420 |
| *Mix (Ragú) *Pizza Quick* | ¼ of pie | 300 |
| **PIZZA PIE CRUST,** refrigerated (Pillsbury) | ⅛ of crust | 90 |
| **PIZZA SAUCE:** | | |
| (Contadina): | | |
| Regular or with cheese | ½ cup | 80 |
| With pepperoni | ½ cup | 90 |
| (Ragú): | | |
| Regular | 2 oz. | 32 |
| *Pizza Quick* | 2 oz. | 45 |
| **PLUM:** | | |
| Fresh, Japanese & hybrid | 2″ dia. | 27 |
| Fresh, prune-type, halves | ½ cup | 60 |
| Canned, regular pack: | | |
| (Stokely-Van Camp) | ½ cup | 120 |
| (Thank You Brand) heavy syrup | ½ cup | 109 |
| Canned, unsweetened, purple, solids & liq.: | | |
| (Diet Delight) juice pack | ½ cup | 70 |
| (Featherweight) water pack | ½ cup | 40 |
| (S&W) *Nutradiet,* juice pack | ½ cup | 80 |
| **PLUM JELLY,** sweetened (Home Brands) | 1 T. | 52 |
| **PLUM PRESERVE OR JAM,** sweetened (Bama) | 1 T. | 45 |
| **PLUM PUDDING** (Richardson & Robbins) | 2″ wedge | 270 |
| **POLYNESIAN-STYLE DINNER,** frozen (Swanson) | 12-oz. dinner | 360 |
| **POMEGRANATE,** whole | 1 lb. | 160 |
| ***PONDEROSA RESTAURANT:*** | | |
| *A-1 Sauce* | 1 tsp. | 4 |
| Beef, chopped (patty only): | | |
| Regular | 3½ oz. | 209 |
| Double Deluxe | 5.9 oz. | 362 |
| Junior (*Square Shooter*) | 1.6 oz. | 98 |
| Steakhouse Deluxe | 2.96 oz. | 181 |
| Beverages: | | |
| *Coca-Cola* | 8 fl. oz. | 96 |
| Coffee | 6 fl. oz. | 2 |
| *Dr. Pepper* | 8 fl. oz. | 96 |
| Milk, chocolate | 8 fl. oz. | 208 |
| Orange drink | 8 fl. oz. | 110 |
| Root beer | 8 fl. oz. | 104 |

| Food and Description | Measure or Quantity | Calories |
|---|---|---|
| *Sprite* | 8 fl. oz. | 95 |
| *Tab* | 8 fl. oz. | 1 |
| Bun: | | |
| Regular | 2.4-oz. bun | 190 |
| Hot dog | 1 bun | 108 |
| Junior | 1.4-oz. bun | 118 |
| Steakhouse deluxe | 2.4-oz. bun | 190 |
| Chicken strips: | | |
| Adult portion | 2¾ oz. | 282 |
| Child | 1.4 oz. | 141 |
| Cocktail sauce | 1½ oz. | 57 |
| Filet mignon | 3.8 oz. (edible portion) | 57 |
| Filet of sole, fish only (See also Bun: regular) | 3-oz. piece | 125 |
| Fish, baked | 4.9-oz. serving | 268 |
| Gelatin dessert | ½ cup | 97 |
| Gravy, au jus | 1 oz. | 3 |
| Ham & cheese: | | |
| Bun (see Bun) | | |
| Cheese, Swiss | 2 slices (.8 oz.) | 76 |
| Ham | 2½ oz. | 184 |
| Hot dog, child's, meat only (see also Bun) | 1.6-oz. hot dog | 140 |
| Margarine: | | |
| Pat | 1 tsp. | 36 |
| On potato, as served | ½ oz. | 100 |
| Mustard sauce, sweet & sour | 1 oz. | 50 |
| New York strip steak | 6.1 oz. (edible portion) | 362 |
| Onion, chopped | 1 T. | 4 |
| Pickle, dill | 3 slices (.7 oz.) | 2 |
| Potato: | | |
| Baked | 7.2-oz. potato | 145 |
| French fries | 3-oz. serving | 230 |
| Prime ribs: | | |
| Regular | 4.2 oz. (edible portion) | 286 |
| King | 6 oz. (edible portion) | 409 |
| Pudding, chocolate | 4½ oz. | 213 |
| Ribeye | 3.2 oz. (edible portion) | 197 |
| Ribeye & shrimp: | | |
| Ribeye | 3.2 oz. | 197 |
| Shrimp | 2.2 oz. | 139 |
| Roll, kaiser | 2.2-oz. roll | 184 |
| Salad bar: | | |
| Bean sprouts | 1 oz. | 13 |

| Food and Description | Measure or Quantity | Calories |
|---|---|---|
| Broccoli | 1 oz. | 9 |
| Cabbage, red | 1 oz. | 9 |
| Carrots | 1 oz. | 12 |
| Cauliflower | 1 oz. | 8 |
| Celery | 1 oz. | 4 |
| Chickpeas (Garbanzos) | 1 oz. | 102 |
| Mushrooms | 1 oz. | 8 |
| Pepper, green | 1 oz. | 6 |
| Radish | 1 oz. | 5 |
| Tomato | 1 oz. | 6 |
| Salad dressing: | | |
| Blue cheese | 1 oz. | 129 |
| Italian, creamy | 1 oz. | 138 |
| Low calorie | 1 oz. | 14 |
| Oil & vinegar | 1 oz. | 124 |
| Thousand Island | 1 oz. | 117 |
| Shrimp dinner | 7 pieces (3½ oz.) | 220 |
| Sirloin: | | |
| Regular | 3.3 oz. (edible portion) | 220 |
| Super | 6½ oz. (edible portion) | 383 |
| Tips | 4 oz. (edible portion) | 192 |
| Steak sauce | 1 oz. | 23 |
| Tartar sauce | 1.5 oz. | 285 |
| T-Bone | 4.3 oz. (edible portion) | 240 |
| Tomato (See also Salad bar): | | |
| Slices | 2 slices (.9 oz.) | 5 |
| Whole, small | 3.5 oz. | 22 |
| Topping, whipped | ¼ oz. | 19 |
| Worcestershire sauce | 1 tsp. | 4 |
| **POPCORN:** | | |
| *Plain, popped fresh: | | |
| (Jiffy Pop) | ½ of 5-oz. pkg. | 244 |
| (Jolly Time) microwave: | | |
| Natural or butter flavor | 1 cup | 53 |
| Cheese flavor | 1 cup | 60 |
| (Orville Reddenbacher's): | | |
| Original: | | |
| Plain | 1 cup | 22 |
| With oil & salt | 1 cup | 40 |
| Caramel crunch | 1 oz. | 140 |
| Hot air popped | 1 cup | 25 |
| Microwave: | | |
| Regular: | | |
| Butter flavored | 1 cup | 27 |
| Natural | 1 cup | 27 |

| Food and Description | Measure or Quantity | Calories |
|---|---|---|
| Flavored: | | |
| Caramel | 1 cup | 96 |
| Cheese, cheddar | 1 cup | 50 |
| Frozen | 1 cup | 35 |
| (Pillsbury) Microwave Popcorn: | | |
| Regular | 1 cup | 70 |
| Butter flavor | 1 cup | 65 |
| *Pop Secret* (General Mills) | 1 cup | 140 |
| Packaged: | | |
| Buttered (Wise) | ½ oz. | 70 |
| Caramel-coated: | | |
| (Bachman) | 1-oz. serving | 130 |
| (Old Dutch) | 1 oz. | 109 |
| (Old London) without peanuts | 1¾-oz. serving | 195 |
| Cheese flavored (Bachman) | 1-oz. serving | 180 |
| *Cracker Jack* | 1-oz. serving | 120 |
| **POPCORN POPPING OIL** (Orville Reddenbacher's) buttery flavor | 1 T. | 120 |
| ***POPOVER MIX** (Flako) | 1 popover | 170 |
| **POPPY SEED** (French's) | 1 tsp. | 13 |
| *POPSICLE*, twin pop | 3 fl. oz. | 70 |
| *POP TARTS* (See TOASTER CAKE OR PASTRY) | | |
| **PORK:** | | |
| Fresh: | | |
| Chop: | | |
| Broiled, lean & fat | 3-oz. chop (weighed without bone) | 332 |
| Broiled, lean only | 3-oz. chop (weighed without bone) | 230 |
| Loin: | | |
| Roasted, lean & fat | 3 oz. | 308 |
| Roasted, lean only | 3 oz. | 216 |
| Spareribs, braised | 3 oz. | 246 |
| Cured ham: | | |
| Roasted, lean & fat | 3 oz. | 246 |
| Roasted, lean only | 3 oz. | 159 |
| **PORK DINNER:** frozen (Swanson) | 11¼-oz. dinner | 290 |
| **PORK DINNER OR ENTREE:** | | |
| Canned (Hunt's) *Minute Gourmet Microwave Entree Maker,* cajun: | | |
| Without pork | 3.9 oz. | 180 |
| *With pork | 6.6 oz. | 460 |
| Frozen (Swanson) dinner, loin of | 11¼-oz. dinner | 290 |
| **PORK, PACKAGED** (Eckrich) | 1-oz. serving | 45 |
| **PORK RINDS** (Tom's) | .6 oz. serving | 60 |
| **PORK STEAK, BREADED,** frozen (Hormel) | 3-oz. serving | 223 |

| Food and Description | Measure or Quantity | Calories |
|---|---|---|
| **PORK, SWEET & SOUR,** frozen | | |
| (La Choy) | ½ of 15-oz. pkg. | 229 |
| **PORT WINE:** | | |
| (Gallo) | 3 fl. oz. | 94 |
| (Louis M. Martini) | 3 fl. oz. | 82 |
| ***POSTUM,*** instant | 6 fl. oz. | 11 |
| **POTATO:** | | |
| Cooked: | | |
| Au gratin | ½ cup | 127 |
| Baked, peeled | 2½"-dia. potato | 92 |
| Boiled, peeled | 4.2-oz. potato | 79 |
| French-fried | 10 pieces | 156 |
| Hash-browned, home recipe | ½ cup | 223 |
| Mashed, milk & butter added | ½ cup | 92 |
| Canned, solids & liq.: | | |
| (Allen's) *Butterfield* | ½ cup | 45 |
| (Del Monte) | ½ cup (4 oz.) | 45 |
| (Larsen) *Freshlike*, sliced or whole | ½ cup (4.5 oz.) | 61 |
| Frozen: | | |
| (Birds Eye): | | |
| Cottage fries | 2.8-oz. serving | 119 |
| Crinkle cuts, regular | 3-oz. serving | 115 |
| Farm style wedge | 3-oz. serving | 109 |
| French fries, regular | 3-oz. serving | 113 |
| Hash browns, shredded | ¼ of 12-oz. pkg. | 61 |
| Steak fries | 3-oz. serving | 109 |
| *Tasti Puffs* | ¼ of 10-oz. pkg. | 192 |
| *Tiny Taters* | ⅕ of 16-oz. pkg. | 204 |
| Whole, peeled | 3.2 oz. | 59 |
| (Empire Kosher) french fries | 3 oz. | 110 |
| (Larsen) diced | 4 oz. | 80 |
| (Stouffer's): | | |
| Au gratin | ⅓ pkg. | 110 |
| Scalloped | ⅓ pkg. | 90 |
| **POTATO & BACON,** canned | | |
| (Hormel) *Short Orders*, au gratin | 7½-oz. can | 240 |
| **POTATO & BEEF,** canned, | | |
| *Dinty Moore* (Hormel) *Short Orders* | 1½-oz. can | 250 |
| **POTATO & HAM,** canned (Hormel) | | |
| *Short Orders*, scalloped | 7½-oz. can | 250 |
| **POTATO CHIP:** | | |
| (Cottage Fries) unsalted | 1 oz. | 160 |
| *Delta Gold,* any style | 1 oz. | 160 |
| (Frito-Lay's) natural | 1 oz. | 157 |
| (Laura Scudder's) | 1 oz. | 150 |
| *Lay's*, sour cream & onion flavor | 1 oz. | 160 |
| (New York Deli) | 1 oz. | 160 |
| *O'Grady's* | 1 oz. | 150 |

134

| Food and Description | Measure or Quantity | Calories |
|---|---|---|
| (Old Dutch): | | |
| Regular or onion & garlic | 1 oz. | 150 |
| BBQ | 1 oz. | 140 |
| *Pringle's:* | | |
| Regular or *Cheez-Ums* | 1 oz. | 167 |
| Light | 1 oz. | 148 |
| (Snyder's) | 1 oz. | 150 |
| *Ruffles*, light | 1 oz. | 130 |
| (Tom's) any type | 1 oz. | 160 |
| (Wise): | | |
| Barbecue or garlic & onion | 1 oz. | 150 |
| Lightly salted, natural or salt & vinegar | 1 oz. | 160 |
| **\*POTATO MIX:** | | |
| Au gratin: | | |
| (Betty Crocker) | ½ cup | 150 |
| (French's) tangy | ½ cup | 130 |
| (Lipton) & sauce | ¼ pkg. | 108 |
| Casserole (French's) | ½ cup | 130 |
| Cheddar bacon (Lipton) & sauce | ½ cup | 106 |
| Cheddar broccoli (Lipton) | ½ cup | 104 |
| Chicken flavored mushroom (Lipton) & sauce | ¼ pkg. | 90 |
| Chicken & herb (Betty Crocker) | ½ cup | 120 |
| Creamed (Betty Crocker) parsley | ½ cup | 180 |
| Hash browns (Betty Crocker) with onion | ½ cup | 160 |
| Italian (Lipton) | ½ cup | 107 |
| Julienne (Betty Crocker) with mild cheese sauce | ½ cup | 140 |
| Mashed: | | |
| (Betty Crocker) *Buds* | ½ cup | 130 |
| (French's) | ½ cup | 140 |
| Nacho (Lipton) & sauce | ½ cup | 103 |
| Scalloped: | | |
| (Betty Crocker) | ½ cup | 140 |
| (Libby's) *Potato Classics* | ¾ cup | 130 |
| (Lipton) & sauce | ¼ cup | 102 |
| Sour cream & chive (Betty Crocker) | ½ cup | 160 |
| Stroganoff (French's) creamy | ½ cup | 130 |
| **\*POTATO PANCAKE MIX** | | |
| (French's) | 3" pancake | 30 |
| **POTATO SALAD:** | | |
| Home recipe | ½ cup | 181 |
| Canned (Nalley's) German style | 4-oz. serving | 143 |
| *Mix: | | |
| (Betty Crocker) | ⅙ of pkg. | 250 |
| (Lipton) German | ½ cup | 99 |

| Food and Description | Measure or Quantity | Calories |
|---|---|---|
| **POTATO STARCH** | | |
| (Manischewitz) pure | ½ cup | 315 |
| **POTATO STICKS** (Durkee) *O & C* | 1½-oz. can | 231 |
| **POTATO, STUFFED, BAKED,** | | |
| frozen (Green Giant): | | |
| With cheese flavored topping | ½ of 10-oz. pkg. | 200 |
| With sour cream & chives | ½ of 10-oz. pkg. | 230 |
| *POTATO TOPPERS* (Libby's) | 1 T. | 30 |
| **POT ROAST,** frozen | | |
| (Stouffer's) *Right Course* | 9¼-oz. meal | 220 |
| **POUND CAKE** (See CAKE, Pound) | | |
| **PRESERVE OR JAM** (See individual | | |
| flavors) | | |
| **PRETZEL:** | | |
| (Eagle Snacks) | 1 oz. | 110 |
| (Estee) unsalted | 1 piece | 5 |
| *Mister Salty:* | | |
| Regular: | | |
| Dutch | .5-oz. piece | 55 |
| Logs | .1-oz. piece | 12 |
| Nuggets | 1 piece | 5 |
| Rods | .5-oz. piece | 55 |
| Stick, *Veri-thin* | 1 piece | 2 |
| Juniors: | 1 piece | 4 |
| (Nabisco) *Mister Salty:* | | |
| Dutch | 1 piece | 55 |
| Mini | 1 piece | 7 |
| Nuggets | 1 piece | 5 |
| Twists | 1 piece | 22 |
| (Rokeach) | 1 oz. | 110 |
| *Rold Gold* | 1 oz. | 110 |
| (Snyder's) hard | 1 oz. | 102 |
| (Tom's) twists | 1 oz. | 100 |
| (Wise) nugget | 1 oz. | 110 |
| *PRODUCT 19,* cereal (Kellogg's) | 1 cup | 100 |
| *PRO GRAIN,* cereal (Kellogg's) | ¾ cup | 100 |
| **PROSCIUTTO** (Hormel) boneless | 1 oz. | 90 |
| **PRUNE:** | | |
| Canned: | | |
| (Featherweight) stewed, | | |
| water pack | ½ cup | 130 |
| (Sunsweet) stewed | ½ cup | 120 |
| Dried: | | |
| (Del Monte) Moist Pak | 2 oz. | 120 |
| (Sunsweet) whole | 2 oz. | 130 |
| **PRUNE JUICE:** | | |
| (Algood) *Lady Betty* | 6 fl. oz. | 130 |
| (Ardmore Farms) | 6 fl. oz. | 148 |

| Food and Description | Measure or Quantity | Calories |
|---|---|---|
| (Del Monte) | 6 fl. oz. | 120 |
| (Mott's) regular | 6 fl. oz. | 140 |
| (Sunsweet) regular | 6 fl. oz. | 140 |
| **PRUNE NECTAR,** canned (Mott's) | 6 fl. oz. | 100 |
| **PUDDING OR PIE FILLING:** | | |
| Canned, regular pack: | | |
| Banana: | | |
| (Del Monte) *Pudding Cup* | 5-oz. container | 181 |
| (Hunt's) *Snack Pack* | 4¼-oz. container | 180 |
| (Thank You Brand) | ½ cup | 150 |
| Butterscotch: | | |
| (Del Monte) *Pudding Cup* | 5-oz. container | 184 |
| (Swiss Miss) | 4-oz. container | 160 |
| (Thank You Brand) | ½ cup | 149 |
| Chocolate: | | |
| (Del Monte) *Pudding Cup* | 5-oz. container | 201 |
| (Hunt's) *Snack Pack:* | | |
| Regular | 4¼-oz. container | 160 |
| Fudge | 4¼-oz. container | 170 |
| Marshmallow | 4¼-oz. container | 190 |
| (Swiss Miss) fudge or fruit on bottom | 4-oz. container | 170 |
| (Thank You Brand) | ½ cup | 191 |
| Rice (Comstock; Menner's) | ½ of 7½-oz. can | 120 |
| Tapioca: | | |
| (Del Monte) *Pudding Cup* | 5-oz. container | 172 |
| (Hunt's) *Snack Pack* | 4¼-oz. container | 160 |
| Vanilla (Del Monte) | 5-oz. container | 188 |
| Canned, dietetic pack: | | |
| (Estee) | ½ cup | 70 |
| (Sego) | 4-oz. serving | 125 |
| Chilled, *Swiss Miss:* | | |
| Butterscotch, chocolate malt or vanilla | 4-oz. container | 150 |
| Chocolate or double rich | 4-oz. container | 160 |
| Tapioca | 4-oz. container | 130 |
| Frozen (Rich's): | | |
| Butterscotch | 4½-oz. container | 198 |
| Chocolate | 4½-oz. container | 212 |
| *Mix, sweetened, regular & instant: | | |
| Banana: | | |
| (Jello-O) cream, regular | ½ cup | 161 |
| (Royal) regular | ½ cup | 160 |
| Butter pecan (Jello-O) instant | ½ cup | 175 |
| Butterscotch: | | |
| (Jell-O) instant | ½ cup | 175 |
| (My-T-Fine) regular | ½ cup | 143 |
| Chocolate | | |
| (Jell-O) regular | ½ cup | 174 |

137

| Food and Description | Measure or Quantity | Calories |
|---|---|---|
| (My-T-Fine) regular | ½ cup | 169 |
| Coconut: | | |
| (Jell-O) cream, regular | ½ cup | 176 |
| (Royal) instant | ½ cup | 170 |
| Flan (Royal) regular | ½ cup | 150 |
| Lemon: | | |
| (Jell-O) instant | ½ cup | 170 |
| (My-T-Fine) regular | ½ cup | 164 |
| Lime (Royal) Key Lime, regular | ½ cup | 160 |
| Pineapple (Jell-O) cream, instant | ½ cup | 176 |
| Pistachio (Jell-O) instant | ½ cup | 174 |
| Raspberry (Salada) | | |
| *Danish Dessert* | ½ cup | 176 |
| Rice, *Jell-O Americana* | ½ cup | 176 |
| Strawberry (Salada) | | |
| *Danish Dessert* | ½ cup | 130 |
| Tapioca: | | |
| *Jell-O Americana,* chocolate | ½ cup | 173 |
| (My-T-Fine) vanilla | ½ cup | 130 |
| Vanilla: | | |
| (Jell-O) French, regular | ½ cup | 172 |
| (Royal) | ½ cup | 180 |
| *Mix, dietetic: | | |
| Butterscotch: | | |
| (D-Zerta) | ½ cup | 68 |
| (Estee) | ½ cup | 70 |
| (Featherweight) artificially sweetened | ½ cup | 60 |
| (Royal) instant | ½ cup | 100 |
| Chocolate: | | |
| (Estee) | ½ cup | 70 |
| (Royal) instant | ½ cup | 100 |
| Lemon (Estee) | ½ cup | 106 |
| Vanilla: | | |
| (D-Zerta) | ½ cup | 71 |
| (Estee) | ½ cup | 70 |
| (Featherweight) artifically sweetened | ½ cup | 60 |
| **PUDDING ROLL-UPS,** (General Mills) *Fruit Corners* | .5-oz. roll | 60 |
| **PUDDING STIX** (Good Humor) | 1¾-fl.-oz. pop | 90 |
| **PUDDING SUNDAE** (Swiss Miss): | | |
| Caramel or mint | 4-oz. container | 170 |
| Chocolate | 4-oz. container | 190 |
| Peanut butter | 4-oz. container | 200 |
| **PUFFED RICE:** | | |
| (Malt-O-Meal) | 1 cup | 50 |
| (Quaker) | 1 cup | 55 |

| Food and Description | Measure or Quantity | Calories |
|---|---|---|
| **PUFFED WHEAT:** | | |
| (Malt-O-Meal) | 1 cup | 50 |
| (Quaker) | 1 cup | 54 |
| **PUMPKIN,** canned (Libby's) | | |
| solid pack | ½ cup | 80 |
| **PUMPKIN SEED,** in hull | 1 oz. | 116 |

# Q

| Food and Description | Measure or Quantity | Calories |
|---|---|---|
| **QUAIL,** raw, meat & skin | 4 oz. | 195 |
| *QUIK,* (Nestlé) chocolate or strawberry | 1 tsp. | 45 |
| *QUISP,* cereal | 1⅙ cup | 121 |

# R

| Food and Description | Measure or Quantity | Calories |
|---|---|---|
| **RADISH** | 2 small radishes | 4 |
| **RAISIN,** dried: | | |
| (Del Monte) golden | 3 oz. | 260 |
| (Sun-Maid) | 1 oz. | 96 |
| *RAISIN SQUARES,* cereal | | |
| (Kellogg's) | ½ cup | 90 |
| *RALSTON,* cereal | ¼ cup | 90 |
| **RASPBERRY:** | | |
| Fresh: | | |
| Black, trimmed | ½ cup | 49 |
| Red, trimmed | ½ cup | 41 |
| Frozen (Birds Eye) quick thaw | 5-oz. serving | 155 |
| **RASPBERRY PRESERVE OR JAM:** | | |
| Sweetened (Smucker's) | 1 T. | 53 |
| Dietetic: | | |
| (Estee, Louis Sherry) | 1 T. | 6 |
| (Featherweight) red | 1 T. | 16 |
| (S&W) *Nutradiet,* red | 1 T. | 12 |
| **RATATOUILLE,** frozen (Stouffer's) | 5-oz. serving | 60 |
| **RAVIOLI:** | | |
| Canncd, regular pack (Franco-American) beef, *RavioliOs* | 7½-oz. serving | 210 |
| Canned, dietetic (Estee) beef | 8-oz. can | 230 |
| Frozen: | | |
| (Buitoni): | | |
| Cheese: | | |
| Regular, square | 4.8 oz. | 331 |
| Ravioletti | 2.6 oz. | 221 |
| Meat, square | 4.8 oz. | 318 |
| (Celantano): | | |
| Regular | 6½ oz. | 410 |
| Mini | 4 oz. | 250 |
| (Weight Watchers) baked | 8-1/16 oz. meal | 290 |
| **RED LOBSTER RESTAURANTS** ("Lunch Portion" refers to a cooked serving weighing 5 oz. raw, unless otherwise noted): | | |
| Calamari, breaded & fried | Lunch portion | 360 |

| Food and Description | Measure or Quantity | Calories |
|---|---|---|
| Catfish | Lunch portion | 170 |
| Chicken breast | 4-oz. serving | 120 |
| Clam, cherrystone | Lunch portion | 130 |
| Cod, Atlantic | Lunch portion | 100 |
| Crab legs: | | |
| King | 16-oz. serving | 170 |
| Snow | 16-oz. serving | 150 |
| Flounder | Lunch portion | 100 |
| Grouper | Lunch portion | 110 |
| Haddock | Lunch portion | 100 |
| Halibut | Lunch portion | 110 |
| Hamburger, without bun | 5.3 oz. | 320 |
| Lobster: | | |
| Maine | 1 lobster (edible portion) | 240 |
| Rock | 1 tail | 230 |
| Mackerel | Lunch portion | 190 |
| Monkfish | Lunch portion | 110 |
| Mussels | 3-oz. serving | 70 |
| Oysters | 6 raw oysters | 110 |
| Perch, Atlantic Ocean | Lunch portion | 130 |
| Pollock | Lunch portion | 120 |
| Rockfish, red | Lunch portion | 90 |
| Salmon: | | |
| Norwegian | Lunch portion | 230 |
| Sockeye | Lunch portion | 160 |
| Scallop: | | |
| Calico | Lunch portion | 180 |
| Deep sea | Lunch portion | 130 |
| Shark: | | |
| Blacktip | Lunch portion | 150 |
| Mako | Lunch portion | 140 |
| Shrimp | 8–12 pieces | 120 |
| Snapper, red | Lunch portion | 110 |
| Sole, lemon | Lunch portion | 120 |
| Steak: | | |
| Porterhouse | 18-oz. serving | 1420 |
| Sirloin | 7-oz. serving | 570 |
| Strip | 7-oz. serving | 690 |
| Swordfish | Lunch portion | 100 |
| Tilefish | Lunch portion | 100 |
| Trout, rainbow | Lunch portion | 170 |
| Tuna, yellowfin | Lunch portion | 180 |
| **RELISH:** | | |
| Dill (Vlasic) | 1 oz. | 2 |
| Hamburger: | | |
| (Heinz) | 1 oz. | 30 |
| (Vlasic) | 1 T. | 24 |

| Food and Description | Measure or Quantity | Calories |
|---|---|---|
| Hot dog: | | |
| (Heinz) | 1 oz. | 35 |
| (Vlasic) | 1 T. | 28 |
| Sweet (Vlasic) | 1 T. | 18 |
| **RENNET MIX** (Junket): | | |
| *Powder, any flavor: | | |
| Made with skim milk | ½ cup | 90 |
| Made with whole milk | ½ cup | 120 |
| Tablet | 1 tablet | 1 |
| **RHINE WINE:** | | |
| (Great Western) | 3 fl. oz. | 73 |
| (Taylor) | 3 fl. oz. | 75 |
| **RHUBARB,** cooked, sweetened | ½ cup | 169 |
| ***RICE:** | | |
| Brown (Uncle Ben's) parboiled, with added butter | ⅔ cup | 152 |
| White: | | |
| (Minute Rice) instant, no added butter | ⅔ cup | 120 |
| (Success) long grain | ½ cooking bag | 110 |
| White & wild (Carolina) | ½ cup | 90 |
| **RICE CAKE** (Pritikin) | 1 cake | 35 |
| **RICE, FRIED** (See also RICE MIX): | | |
| *Canned (La Choy) | ¾ cup | 180 |
| Frozen: | | |
| (Birds Eye) | 3.7-oz. serving | 104 |
| (Chun King) pork | 8 oz. | 263 |
| (La Choy) & meat | 8-oz. serving | 280 |
| **RICE, FRIED, SEASONING MIX** | | |
| (Kikkoman) | 1-oz. pkg. | 91 |
| *RICE KRINKLES,* cereal (Post) | ⅞ cup | 109 |
| *RICE KRISPIES,* cereal (Kellogg's): | | |
| Regular, frosted, cocoa or strawberry | 1 oz. | 110 |
| Marshmallow | 1 oz. | 140 |
| **RICE MIX:** | | |
| Beef: | | |
| *(Carolina) *Bake-It-Easy* | ¼ pkg. | 110 |
| (Lipton) & sauce | ¼ pkg. | 120 |
| *(Minute Rice) | ½ cup | 149 |
| *Rice-A-Roni* | ⅙ pkg. | 130 |
| *Cajun (Lipton) & sauce | ¼ pkg. | 123 |
| Chicken: | | |
| *(Carolina) *Bake-It-Easy* | ¼ pkg. | 110 |
| (Lipton) & sauce | ¼ pkg. | 125 |
| *Rice-A-Roni* | ⅙ pkg. | 130 |
| *Fried (Minute Rice) | ½ cup | 160 |
| Herb & butter (Lipton) & sauce | ¼ pkg. | 124 |
| *Long grain & wild (Minute Rice) | ½ cup | 150 |
| Mushroom (Lipton) & sauce | ¼ pkg. | 123 |

| Food and Description | Measure or Quantity | Calories |
|---|---|---|
| *Oriental (Carolina) *Bake-It-Easy* | ½ pkg. | 120 |
| *Pilaf (Lipton) & sauce | ½ cup | 117 |
| Spanish: | | |
| *(Carolina) *Bake-It-Easy* | ¼ pkg. | 110 |
| *(Lipton) & sauce | ½ cup | 120 |
| *Rice-A-Roni* | ⅓ pkg. | 110 |
| **\*RICE SEASONING** (French's) | | |
| *Spice Your Rice:* | | |
| Beef flavor & onion or | | |
| cheese & chives | ½ cup | 160 |
| Buttery herb | ½ cup | 170 |
| **RICE, SPANISH:** | | |
| Canned: | | |
| Regular pack (Comstock; | | |
| Menner's) | ½ of 7½-oz. can | 140 |
| Dietetic (Featherweight) | | |
| low sodium | 7½-oz. serving | 140 |
| Frozen (Birds Eye) | 3.7-oz. serving | 122 |
| **RICE & VEGETABLE,** frozen: | | |
| (Birds Eye): | | |
| For One: | | |
| & broccoli, au gratin | 5-oz. pkg. | 229 |
| Mexican, with corn | 5½-oz. pkg. | 158 |
| International: | | |
| Country style | ⅓ of pkg. | 87 |
| Spanish style | ⅓ of pkg. | 111 |
| (Green Giant) *Rice Originals* | | |
| & broccoli in cheese sauce | 4 oz. | 120 |
| Pilaf | 4 oz. | 130 |
| **RICE WINE:** | | |
| Chinese, 20.7% alcohol | 1 fl. oz. | 38 |
| Japanese, 10.6% alcohol | 1 fl. oz. | 72 |
| **ROCK & RYE** (Mr. Boston) | 1 fl. oz. | 75 |
| ***ROCKY ROAD,*** cereal (General Mills) | ⅔ cup | 120 |
| **ROE,** baked or broiled, cod & shad | 4 oz. | 143 |
| **ROLL OR BUN:** | | |
| Commercial type, non-frozen: | | |
| Biscuit (Wonder) | 1¼-oz. piece | 80 |
| Brown & serve (Wonder) | | |
| *Gem Style* | 1-oz. piece | 80 |
| Cherry (Dolly Madison) | 2-oz. piece | 180 |
| Cinnamon (Dolly Madison) | 1¾-oz. piece | 180 |
| Club (Pepperidge Farm) | 1.3-oz. piece | 100 |
| Crescent (Pepperidge Farm) | | |
| butter | 1-oz. piece | 110 |
| Croissant (Pepperidge Farm): | | |
| Butter, cinnamon or | | |
| honey-sesame | 2-oz. piece | 200 |
| Chocolate | 2.4-oz. piece | 260 |

144

| Food and Description | Measure or Quantity | Calories |
|---|---|---|
| Walnut | 2-oz. piece | 210 |
| Danish (Dolly Madison) | | |
| *Danish Twirls:* | | |
| Apple | 2-oz. piece | 240 |
| Cheese, cream | 3½-oz. piece | 380 |
| Cinnamon raisin | 2-oz. piece | 250 |
| Dinner: | | |
| *Butternut* (Interstate Brands) | 1-oz. roll | 90 |
| *Home Pride* | 1-oz. piece | 85 |
| (Pepperidge Farm) | .7-oz. piece | 60 |
| Finger (Pepperidge Farm) sesame or poppy seed | .6-oz. piece | 60 |
| Frankfurter: | | |
| (Arnold) Hot Dog | 1.3-oz. piece | 100 |
| (Pepperidge Farm) | 1¾-oz. piece | 110 |
| (Wonder) | 1-oz. piece | 80 |
| French: | | |
| (Arnold) *Francisco,* sourdough | 1.1-oz. piece | 90 |
| (Pepperidge Farm): | | |
| Small | 1.3-oz. piece | 110 |
| Large | 3-oz. piece | 240 |
| *Golden Twist* (Pepperidge Farm) | 1-oz. piece | 110 |
| Hamburger: | | |
| (Arnold) | 1.4-oz. piece | 110 |
| (Pepperidge Farm) | 1.5-oz. piece | 130 |
| *Roman Meal* | 1.8-oz. piece | 193 |
| Hoagie (Wonder) | 5-oz. piece | 400 |
| Honey (Dolly Madison) | 3½-oz. piece | 420 |
| Kaiser (Interstate Brands): | | |
| *Dutch Hearth* | 1½-oz. piece | 110 |
| *Sweetheart* | 2-oz. piece | 150 |
| Lemon (Dolly Madison) | 2-oz. piece | 180 |
| Old fashioned (Pepperidge Farm) | .6-oz. piece | 60 |
| Parkerhouse (Pepperidge Farm) | .6-oz. piece | 50 |
| Party (Pepperidge Farm) | .4-oz. piece | 30 |
| Raspberry (Dolly Madison) | 2-oz. piece | 190 |
| Sandwich (Arnold) soft | 1.3-oz. piece | 110 |
| Soft (Pepperidge Farm) | 1¼-oz. piece | 110 |
| Frozen: | | |
| Apple crunch (Sara Lee) | 1-oz. piece | 102 |
| Caramel pecan (Sara Lee) | 1.3-oz. piece | 161 |
| Cinnamon (Sara Lee) | .9-oz. piece | 100 |
| Croissant (Sara Lee) | .9-oz. piece | 109 |
| Crumb (Sara Lee) French | 1¾-oz. piece | 188 |
| Danish (Sara Lee): | | |
| Apple | 1.3-oz. piece | 120 |
| Cheese | 1.3-oz. piece | 130 |
| Cinnamon raisin | 1.3-oz. piece | 147 |
| Pecan | 1.3-oz. piece | 148 |

| Food and Description | Measure or Quantity | Calories |
|---|---|---|
| Honey (Morton) mini | 1.3-oz. piece | 133 |
| **\*ROLL OR BUN DOUGH:** | | |
| Frozen (Rich's) home style | 1 piece | 75 |
| Refrigerated (Pillsbury): | | |
| Caramel danish, with nuts | 1 piece | 160 |
| Cinnamon raisin danish | 1 piece | 110 |
| Crescent | 1 piece | 100 |
| **\*ROLL MIX, HOT** (Pillsbury) | 1 piece | 120 |
| ***ROMAN MEAL CEREAL*** | ⅓ cup | 103 |
| **ROSEMARY LEAVES** (French's) | 1 tsp. | 5 |
| **ROSÉ WINE:** | | |
| *Corbett Canyon* (Glenmore) | 3 fl. oz. | 63 |
| (Great Western) | 3 fl. oz. | 80 |
| (Paul Masson): | | |
| Regular, 11.8% alcohol | 3 fl. oz. | 76 |
| Light, 7.1% alcohol | 3 fl. oz. | 49 |
| ***ROY ROGERS:*** | | |
| Bar Burger, R.R. | 1 burger | 611 |
| Biscuit | 1 biscuit | 231 |
| Breakfast crescent sandwich: | | |
| Regular | 4.5-oz. sandwich | 401 |
| With bacon | 4.7-oz. sandwich | 431 |
| With ham | 5.8-oz. sandwich | 557 |
| With sausage | 5.7-oz. sandwich | 449 |
| Brownie | 1 piece | 264 |
| Cheeseburger: | | |
| Regular | 1 burger | 563 |
| With bacon | 1 burger | 581 |
| Chicken: | | |
| Breast | 1 piece | 412 |
| Leg | 1 piece | 140 |
| Thigh | 1 piece | 296 |
| Wing | 1 piece | 192 |
| Coleslaw | 3½-oz. serving | 110 |
| Danish: | | |
| Apple | 1 piece | 249 |
| Cheese | 1 piece | 254 |
| Cherry | 1 piece | 271 |
| Drinks: | | |
| Coffee, black | 6 fl. oz. | Tr. |
| Coke: | | |
| Regular | 12 fl. oz. | 145 |
| Diet | 12 fl. oz. | 1 |
| Hot chocolate | 6 fl. oz. | 123 |
| Milk | 8 fl. oz. | 150 |
| Orange juice: | | |
| Regular | 7 fl. oz. | 99 |
| Large | 10 fl. oz. | 136 |

| Food and Description | Measure or Quantity | Calories |
|---|---|---|
| Shake: | | |
| Chocolate | 1 shake | 358 |
| Strawberry | 1 shake | 306 |
| Vanilla | 1 shake | 315 |
| Tea, iced, plain | 8 fl. oz. | 0 |
| Egg & biscuit platter: | | |
| Regular | 1 meal | 394 |
| With bacon | 1 meal | 435 |
| With ham | 1 meal | 442 |
| With sausage | 1 meal | 550 |
| Hamburger | 1 burger | 456 |
| Pancake platter, with syrup & butter | | |
| Plain | 1 order | 452 |
| With bacon | 1 order | 493 |
| With ham | 1 order | 506 |
| With sausage | 1 order | 608 |
| Potato: | | |
| Baked, *Hot Topped:* | | |
| Plain | 1 potato | 211 |
| With bacon & cheese | 1 potato | 397 |
| With broccoli & cheese | 1 potato | 376 |
| With margarine | 1 potato | 274 |
| With sour cream & chives | 1 potato | 408 |
| With taco beef & cheese | 1 potato | 463 |
| French fries: | | |
| Regular | 3 oz. | 268 |
| Large | 4 oz. | 357 |
| Potato salad | 3½-oz. order | 107 |
| Roast beef sandwich: | | |
| Plain: | | |
| Regular | 1 sandwich | 317 |
| Large | 1 sandwich | 360 |
| With cheese: | | |
| Regular | 1 sandwich | 424 |
| Large | 1 sandwich | 467 |
| Salad bar: | | |
| Bacon bits | 1 T. | 33 |
| Beets, sliced | ¼ cup | 16 |
| Broccoli | ½ cup | 20 |
| Carrot, shredded | ¼ cup | 42 |
| Cheese, cheddar | ¼ cup | 112 |
| Croutons | 1 T. | 35 |
| Egg, chopped | 1 T. | 27 |
| Lettuce | 1 cup | 10 |
| Macaroni salad | 1 T. | 30 |
| Mushrooms | ¼ cup | 5 |
| Noodle, Chinese | ¼ cup | 55 |
| Pepper, green | 1 T. | 2 |
| Potato salad | 1 T. | 25 |

| Food and Description | Measure or Quantity | Calories |
|---|---|---|
| Tomato | 1 slice | 7 |
| Salad dressing: | | |
| Regular: | | |
| Bacon & tomato | 1 T. | 68 |
| Bleu cheese | 1 T. | 75 |
| Ranch | 1 T. | 77 |
| 1,000 Island | 1 T. | 80 |
| Low calorie, Italian | 1 T. | 35 |
| Strawberry shortcake | 7.2-oz. serving | 447 |
| Sundae: | | |
| Caramel | 1 sundae | 293 |
| Hot fudge | 1 sundae | 337 |
| Strawberry | 1 sundae | 216 |
| **RUTABAGA:** | | |
| Canned (Sunshine) solids & liq. | ½ cup | 32 |
| Frozen (Sunshine) | 4 oz. | 50 |

# S

| Food and Description | Measure or Quantity | Calories |
|---|---|---|
| **SAFFLOWER SEED,** in hull | 1 oz. | 89 |
| **SAGE** (French's) | 1 tsp. | 4 |
| **SAKE WINE** | 1 fl. oz. | 39 |
| ***SALAD BAR PASTA*** (Buitoni): | | |
|   Country buttermilk | ⅙ of pkg. | 250 |
|   Italian, creamy | ⅙ of pkg. | 290 |
| ***SALAD CRUNCHIES*** (Libby's) | 1 T. | 35 |
| **SALAD DRESSING:** | | |
|   Regular: | | |
|     Bacon (Seven Seas) creamy | 1 T. | 60 |
|     Bacon & tomato (Henri's) | 1 T. | 70 |
|     Bleu or blue cheese | | |
|       (Henri's) | 1 T. | 60 |
|     Caesar: | | |
|       (Pfeiffer) | 1 T. | 70 |
|       (Wish-Bone) | 1 T. | 78 |
|     Capri (Seven Seas) | 1 T. | 70 |
|     Cheddar & bacon (Wish-Bone) | 1 T. | 70 |
|     Cucumber (Wish-Bone) | 1 T. | 80 |
|     French: | | |
|       (Bernstein's) creamy | 1 T. | 56 |
|       (Henri's): | | |
|         Hearty | 1 T. | 70 |
|         Original | 1 T. | 60 |
|       (Seven Seas) creamy | 1 T. | 60 |
|       (Wish-Bone) garlic | 1 T. | 55 |
|     Garlic (Wish-Bone) creamy | 1 T. | 74 |
|     Green Goddess (Seven Seas) | 1 T. | 60 |
|     Herb & spice (Seven Seas) | 1 T. | 60 |
|     Italian: | | |
|       (Bernstein's) | 1 T. | 50 |
|       (Henri's): | | |
|         Authentic | 1 T. | 80 |
|         Creamy garlic | 1 T. | 50 |
|       (Pfeiffer) chef | 1 T. | 60 |
|       (Seven Seas) *Viva!* | 1 T. | 70 |
|       (Wish-Bone) robusto | 1 T. | 70 |
|     Mayonnaise-type, *Blue Plate* | | |
|       (Luzianne) | 1 T. | 70 |

| Food and Description | Measure or Quantity | Calories |
|---|---|---|
| *Miracle Whip* (Kraft) | 1 T. | 70 |
| Ranchouse (Henri's) *Chef's Recipe* | 1 T. | 70 |
| Red wine vinegar & oil (Seven Seas) | 1 T. | 60 |
| Roquefort: | | |
| (Bernstein's) | 1 T. | 65 |
| (Marie's) | 1 T. | 105 |
| Russian: | | |
| (Henri's) | 1 T. | 60 |
| (Pfeiffer) | 1 T. | 65 |
| (Wish-Bone) | 1 T. | 47 |
| Sour cream & bacon (Wish-Bone) | 1 T. | 70 |
| *Spin Blend* (Hellmann's) | 1 T. | 57 |
| *Tas-Tee* (Henri's) | 1 T. | 60 |
| Thousand Island: | | |
| (Pfeiffer) | 1 T. | 65 |
| (Wish-Bone) plain | 1 T. | 61 |
| Vinaigrette (Bernstein's) French | 1 T. | 49 |
| Dietetic or low calorie: | | |
| Bacon & tomato (Estee) | 1 T. | 8 |
| Bleu or blue cheese: | | |
| (Estee) | 1 T. | 8 |
| (Featherweight) imitation | 1 T. | 4 |
| (Herni's) | 1 T. | 35 |
| (Tillie Lewis) *Tasti-Diet* | 1 T. | 12 |
| (Walden Farms) chunky | 1 T. | 27 |
| (Wish-Bone) chunky | 1 T. | 40 |
| Buttermilk (Estee) | 1 T. | 6 |
| Catalina (Kraft) | 1 T. | 16 |
| *Chef's Recipe Ranchouse* (Henri's) | 1 T. | 40 |
| Cucumber (Kraft) | 1 T. | 30 |
| Dijon (Estee) creamy | 1 T. | 8 |
| French: | | |
| (Estee) | 1 T. | 4 |
| (Featherweight) low calorie | 1 T. | 6 |
| (Henri's) original | 1 T. | 40 |
| (Pritikin) | 1 T. | 10 |
| (Walden Farms) | 1 T. | 33 |
| (Wish-Bone) | 1 T. | 31 |
| Herb basket, *Herb Magic* (Luzianne Blue Plate) | 1 T. | 6 |
| Herb & spice (Featherweight) | 1 T. | 6 |
| Garlic (Estee) | 1 T. | 2 |
| Italian: | | |
| (Estee) creamy | 1 T. | 4 |
| (Henri's) hearty | 1 T. | 35 |
| *Herb Magic* (Luzianne Blue Plate) | 1 T. | 4 |
| (Pritikin) creamy | 1 T. | 16 |

| Food and Description | Measure or Quantity | Calories |
|---|---|---|
| (Walden Farms) | 1 T. | 9 |
| (Weight Watchers) | 1 T. | 50 |
| (Wish-Bone) | 1 T. | 7 |
| Olive oil vinaigrette (Wish-Bone) | 1 T. | 16 |
| Onion & chive (Wish-Bone) | 1 T. | 37 |
| Ranch (Pritikin) | 1 T. | 18 |
| Red wine/vinegar (Featherweight) | 1 T. | 6 |
| Russian: | | |
| (Featherweight) creamy | 1 T. | 6 |
| (Pritikin) | 1 T. | 12 |
| (Weight Watchers) | 1 T. | 50 |
| (Wish-Bone) | 1 T. | 25 |
| Sweet & sour, *Herb Magic* | | |
| (Luzianne Blue Plate) | 1 T. | 18 |
| Tas-Tee (Henri's) | 1 T. | 30 |
| Thousand Island: | | |
| (Estee) | 1 T. | 8 |
| (Henri's) | 1 T. | 30 |
| *Herb Magic* (Luzianne Blue | | |
| Plate) | 1 T. | 8 |
| (Kraft) | 1 T. | 30 |
| (Walden Farms) | 1 T. | 24 |
| (Weight Watchers) | 1 T. | 50 |
| (Wish-Bone) | 1 T. | 40 |
| Tomato (Pritikin) zesty | 1 T. | 18 |
| *2-Calorie Low Sodium* | | |
| (Featherweight) | 1 T. | 2 |
| Vinaigrette (Pritikin) | 1 T. | 10 |
| **SALAD DRESSING MIX:** | | |
| *Regular (Good Seasons): | | |
| Blue cheese & herbs | 1 T. | 80 |
| Buttermilk, farm style | 1 T. | 60 |
| Garlic, cheese | 1 T. | 80 |
| Garlic & herb | 1 T. | 80 |
| Italian, regular, cheese or zesty | 1 T. | 80 |
| Dietetic: | | |
| *Blue cheese (Weight Watchers) | 1 T. | 10 |
| *French (Weight Watchers) | 1 T. | 4 |
| Garlic (Dia-Mel) | ½-oz. pkg. | 21 |
| *Italian: | | |
| (Good Seasons) regular | 1 T. | 25 |
| (Weight Watchers): | | |
| Regular | 1 T. | 2 |
| Creamy | 1 T. | 4 |
| *Russian (Weight Watchers) | 1 T. | 4 |
| *Thousand Island | | |
| (Weight Watchers) | 1 T. | 12 |
| **SALAD SUPREME** (McCormick) | 1 tsp. | 11 |

| Food and Description | Measure or Quantity | Calories |
|---|---|---|
| **SALAMI:** | | |
| (Eckrich) for beer or cooked | 1 oz. | 70 |
| *Hebrew National,* beef | 1 oz. | 80 |
| (Hormel): | | |
| Beef | 1 slice | 40 |
| Genoa, DiLusso | 1-oz. serving | 100 |
| Hard, sliced | 1 slice | 34 |
| (Ohse) cooked | 1 oz. | 65 |
| (Oscar Mayer): | | |
| For beer, beef | .8-oz. slice | 64 |
| Cotto | .8-oz. slice | 53 |
| Genoa | .3-oz. slice | 34 |
| **SALISBURY STEAK,** frozen: | | |
| (Armour) *Classic Lite* | 10-oz. meal | 270 |
| (Banquet): | | |
| *Buffet Supper* | 2-lb. pkg. | 1260 |
| *Man Pleaser* | 19-oz. dinner | 1024 |
| (Morton) | 10-oz. meal | 294 |
| (Stouffer's) *Lean Cuisine* | 9½-oz. pkg. | 280 |
| (Swanson): | | |
| Regular: | | |
| Dinner, 4-compartment | 11-oz. dinner | 460 |
| Entree | 5½-oz. entree | 370 |
| *Hungry Man* | 16½-oz. dinner | 710 |
| Main Course | 8½-oz. entree | 430 |
| (Weight Watchers) beef, Romano | 8¾-oz. meal | 300 |
| **SALMON:** | | |
| Baked or broiled | 6¾″ × 2½″ × 1″ piece | 264 |
| Canned, regular pack, solids & liq.: | | |
| Keta (Bumble Bee) | ½ cup | 153 |
| Pink or Humpback: | | |
| (Bumble Bee) | ½ cup | 155 |
| (Del Monte) | 7¾-oz. can | 290 |
| Sockeye or Red or Blueback: | | |
| (Bumble Bee) | ½ cup | 188 |
| (Libby's) | 7¾-oz. can | 380 |
| Canned, dietetic (S&W) *Nutradiet,* low sodium | ½ cup | 188 |
| **SALMON, SMOKED** (Vita): | | |
| Lox, drained | 4-oz. jar | 136 |
| Nova, drained | 4-oz. can | 221 |
| **SALT:** | | |
| (Morton): | | |
| Regular | 1 tsp. | 0 |
| *Lite* | 1 tsp. | 0 |
| Substitute: | | |
| (Adolph's) plain | 1 tsp. | 1 |
| (Morton) plain | 1 tsp. | Tr. |
| *Salt-It* (Estee) | 1 tsp. | 0 |

152

| Food and Description | Measure or Quantity | Calories |
|---|---|---|
| **SALT 'N SPICE SEASONING** | | |
| (McCormick) | 1 tsp. | 3 |
| **SANDWICH SPREAD:** | | |
| (Hellmann's) | 1 T. | 65 |
| (Oscar Mayer) | 1-oz. serving | 67 |
| **SANGRIA** (Taylor) | 3 fl. oz. | 99 |
| **SARDINE,** canned: | | |
| Atlantic (Del Monte) with tomato sauce | 7½-oz. can | 319 |
| Imported (Underwood) in mustard or tomato sauce | 3¾-oz. can | 220 |
| Norwegian: | | |
| (Granadaisa Brand) in tomato sauce | 3¾-oz. can | 195 |
| (King David Brand) brisling in olive oil | 3¾-oz. can | 293 |
| (Queen Helga Brand) in sild oil | 3¾-oz. can | 310 |
| **SAUCE:** | | |
| Regular: | | |
| *A-1* | 1 T. | 12 |
| Barbecue: | | |
| *Chris & Pitt's* | 1 T. | 15 |
| (Gold's) | 1 T. | 25 |
| (Heinz) | ¼ cup | 80 |
| (Hunt's) hickory | 1 T. | 25 |
| (Kraft) plain or hot | ¼ cup | 80 |
| (La Choy) oriental | 1 T. | 16 |
| *Open Pit* (General Foods) original, hot n' spicy or smoke flavor | 1 T. | 25 |
| Burrito (Del Monte) | ¼ cup | 20 |
| Cheese (Snow's) welsh rarebit | ½ cup | 170 |
| Chili (See CHILI SAUCE) | | |
| Cocktail: | | |
| (Gold's) | 1 T. | 31 |
| (Pfeiffer) | 1-oz. serving | 100 |
| *Escoffier Sauce Diable* | 1 T. | 20 |
| *Escoffier Sauce Robert* | 1 T. | 20 |
| *Famous Sauce* | 1 T. | 69 |
| Hot (Gebhardt) | 1 tsp. | 0 |
| Italian (See also SPAGHETTI SAUCE or TOMATO SAUCE): | | |
| (Contadina) | 4-oz. serving | 71 |
| (Ragú) red cooking | 3½-oz. serving | 45 |
| Newberg (Snow's) | ⅓ cup | 120 |
| Orange (La Choy) | 1 T. | 23 |
| Plum (La Choy) tangy | 1 oz. | 44 |
| Salsa Brava (La Victoria) | 1 T. | 6 |
| Salsa Casera (La Victoria) | 1 T. | 4 |
| Salsa Jalapeño (La Victoria) | 1 T. | 4 |

| Food and Description | Measure or Quantity | Calories |
|---|---|---|
| Salsa Mexicana (Contadina) | 4 fl. oz. | 38 |
| Salsa Picante (Del Monte) regular | ¼ cup | 20 |
| Salsa Ranchera (La Victoria) | 1 T. | 6 |
| Salsa Roja (Del Monte) | ¼ cup | 20 |
| Salsa Suprema (La Victoria) | 1 T. | 4 |
| Seafood cocktail (Del Monte) | 1 T. | 21 |
| Soy: | | |
| (Chun King) | 1 T. | 5 |
| (Gold's) | 1 T. | 10 |
| (Kikkoman) light | 1 T. | 11 |
| (La Choy) | 1 T. | Tr. |
| Spare rib (Gold's) | 1 oz. | 60 |
| Sweet & sour: | | |
| (Chun King) | 1.8 oz. | 57 |
| (Contadina) | 4 fl. oz. | 150 |
| (La Choy) | 1 T. | 30 |
| Szechuan (La Choy) | | |
| hot & spicy | 1 oz. | 48 |
| *Tabasco* | ¼ tsp. | Tr. |
| Taco: | | |
| (La Victoria) red | 1 T. | 6 |
| *Old El Paso,* hot or mild | 1 T. | 5 |
| (Ortega) hot or mild | 1 oz. | 13 |
| Tartar: | | |
| (Hellmann's) | 1 T. | 73 |
| (Nalley's) | 1 T. | 89 |
| Teriyaki (Kikkoman) | 1 T. | 15 |
| *V-8* | 1-oz. serving | 25 |
| White, medium | ¼ cup | 103 |
| Worcestershire: | | |
| (French's) regular or smoky | 1 T. | 10 |
| (Gold's) | 1 T. | 42 |
| Dietetic (Estee): | | |
| Barbecue | 1 T. | 18 |
| Cocktail | 1 T. | 10 |
| Taco | 1 oz. | 14 |
| **SAUCE MIX:** | | |
| Regular: | | |
| A la King (Durkee) | 1-oz. pkg. | 133 |
| *Cheese: | | |
| (Durkee) | ½ cup | 168 |
| (French's) | ½ cup | 160 |
| Hollandaise: | | |
| (Durkee) | 1-oz. pkg. | 173 |
| *(French's) | 1 T. | 15 |
| *Sour cream (French's) | 2½ T. | 60 |
| *Sweet & sour (Kikkoman) | 1 T. | 18 |
| Teriyaki (Kikkoman) | 1.5-oz. pkg. | 125 |
| *White (Durkee) | 1 cup | 238 |

| Food and Description | Measure or Quantity | Calories |
|---|---|---|
| *Dietetic (Weight Watchers) lemon butter | 1 T. | 8 |
| **SAUERKRAUT,** canned: | | |
| (Claussen) drained | ½ cup | 16 |
| (Comstock) regular | ½ cup | 30 |
| (Del Monte) solids & liq. | 1 cup | 55 |
| (Silver Floss) solids & liq.: | | |
| Regular | ½ cup | 30 |
| *Krispy Kraut* | ½ cup | 25 |
| (Vlasic) | 2 oz. | 8 |
| **SAUSAGE:** | | |
| *Brown & Serve (Hormel) | 1 sausage | 70 |
| Links (Ohse) hot | 1 oz. | 80 |
| Patty (Hormel) | 1 patty | 150 |
| Polish-style: | | |
| (Eckrich) | 1-oz. serving | 95 |
| (Hormel) *Kilbase* | 1-oz. serving | 122 |
| (Ohse) regular | 1 oz. | 80 |
| Pork: | | |
| (Eckrich) | 1-oz. link | 100 |
| *(Hormel) *Little Sizzlers* | 1 link | 51 |
| (Jimmy Dean) | 2-oz. serving | 227 |
| *(Oscar Mayer) *Little Friers* | 1 link | 79 |
| Roll (Eckrich) minced | 1-oz. slice | 80 |
| Smoked: | | |
| (Eckrich) beef, *Smok-Y-Links* | .8-oz. link | 70 |
| (Hormel) smokies | 1 sausage | 80 |
| (Ohse) | 1 oz. | 80 |
| (Oscar Mayer) beef | 1½-oz. link | 126 |
| *Turkey (Louis Rich) links or tube | 1-oz. serving | 45 |
| Vienna: | | |
| (Hormel) regular | 1 sausage | 50 |
| (Libby's) in barbecue sauce | 2½-oz. serving | 180 |
| **SAUTERNE:** | | |
| (Great Western) | 3 fl. oz. | 79 |
| (Taylor) | 3 fl. oz. | 81 |
| **SCALLOP:** | | |
| Steamed | 4-oz. serving | 127 |
| Frozen: | | |
| (Mrs. Paul's) breaded & fried | 3½-oz. serving | 210 |
| (Stouffer's) *Lean Cuisine* | 11-oz. pkg. | 230 |
| **SCHNAPPS, APPLE** (Mr. Boston) | 1 fl. oz. | 78 |
| **SCHNAPPS, PEPPERMINT** (Mr. Boston) | 1 fl. oz. | 115 |
| **SCREWDRIVER COCKTAIL** (Mr. Boston) 12½% alcohol | 3 fl. oz. | 111 |
| **SCROD DINNER OR ENTREE,** frozen (Gorton's) *Light Recipe* | 1 pkg. | 260 |

| Food and Description | Measure or Quantity | Calories |
|---|---|---|
| **SEAFOOD NEWBERG,** frozen: | | |
| (Armour) *Dinner Classics* | 11½-oz. meal | 300 |
| (Mrs. Paul's) | 8½ oz. | 310 |
| **SEAFOOD PLATTER,** frozen | | |
| (Mrs. Paul's) breaded & fried | 9-oz. serving | 510 |
| *SEGO DIET FOOD,* canned: | | |
| Regular | 10-fl.-oz. can | 225 |
| Lite | 10-fl.-oz. can | 150 |
| *SELTZER* (Canada Dry) | Any quantity | 0 |
| *SERUTAN* | 1 tsp. | 6 |
| **SESAME SEEDS** (French's) | 1 tsp. | 9 |
| **7-GRAIN CEREAL** | | |
| (Loma Linda) | 1 oz. | 110 |
| **SHAD, CREOLE** | 4-oz. serving | 172 |
| *SHAKE 'N BAKE:* | | |
| Chicken, original | 1 pkg. | 320 |
| Fish | 2-oz. pkg. | 280 |
| Italian | 1 pkg. | 320 |
| Pork, barbecue | 1 pkg. | 320 |
| *SHAKEY'S* | | |
| Chicken, fried, & potatoes: | | |
| 3-piece | 1 order | 947 |
| 5-piece | 1 order | 1700 |
| Ham & cheese sandwich | 1 sandwich | 550 |
| Pizza: | | |
| Cheese: | | |
| Thin | 13″ pizza | 1403 |
| Thick | 13″ pizza | 1890 |
| Onion, green pepper, olive & mushroom: | | |
| Thin | 13″ pizza | 1713 |
| Thick | 13″ pizza | 2200 |
| Pepperoni: | | |
| Thin | 13″ pizza | 1833 |
| Thick | 13″ pizza | 2320 |
| Sausage & mushroom: | | |
| Thin | 13″ pizza | 1759 |
| Thick | 13″ pizza | 2256 |
| Sausage & pepperoni: | | |
| Thin | 13″ pizza | 2111 |
| Thick | 13″ pizza | 2598 |
| Special: | | |
| Thin | 13″ pizza | 2110 |
| Thick | 13″ pizza | 2597 |
| Potatoes | 15-piece order | 950 |
| Spaghetti with meat sauce & garlic bread | 1 order | 940 |
| Super hot hero | 1 sandwich | 810 |

| Food and Description | Measure or Quantity | Calories |
|---|---|---|
| **SHELLS, PASTA, STUFFED,** | | |
| frozen: | | |
| (Buitoni) jumbo, cheese stuffed | 5½-oz. serving | 288 |
| (Celentano): | | |
| Broccoli & cheese | 11½-oz. pkg. | 400 |
| Cheese: | | |
| Without sauce | ½ of 12½-oz. pkg. | 350 |
| With sauce | ½ of 16-oz. pkg. | 320 |
| (Stouffer's) cheese stuffed | 9-oz. serving | 320 |
| **SHERBET OR SORBET:** | | |
| Cassis (Häagen-Dazs) | 4 fl. oz. | 128 |
| Daiquiri Ice (Häagen-Dazs) | 4 fl. oz. | 136 |
| Lemon (Häagen-Dazs) | 4 fl. oz. | 140 |
| Orange: | | |
| (Baskin-Robbins) | 4 fl. oz. | 158 |
| (Borden) | ½ cup | 110 |
| (Häagen-Dazs) | 4 fl. oz. | 140 |
| Rainbow (Baskin-Robbins) | 4 fl. oz. | 160 |
| Raspberry: | | |
| (Baskin-Robbins) | 4 fl. oz. | 140 |
| (Sealtest) | ½ cup | 140 |
| **SHERRY:** | | |
| Cocktail (Gold Seal) | 3 fl. oz. | 122 |
| Cream (Great Western) Solera | 3 fl. oz. | 141 |
| Dry (Williams & Humbert) | 3 fl. oz. | 120 |
| Dry Sack (Williams & Humbert) | 3 fl. oz. | 120 |
| **SHREDDED WHEAT:** | | |
| (Nabisco): | | |
| Regular size | ¾-oz. biscuit | 90 |
| *Spoon Size* | ⅔ cup | 110 |
| (Quaker) | 1 biscuit | 52 |
| (Sunshine): | | |
| Regular | 1 biscuit | 90 |
| Bite size | ⅔ cup | 110 |
| **SHRIMP:** | | |
| Canned (Bumble Bee) solids & liq. | 4½-oz. can | 90 |
| Frozen (Mrs. Paul's): | | |
| Breaded & fried | 3 oz. | 190 |
| Parmesan | 11-oz. meal | 310 |
| **SHRIMP & CHICKEN CANTONESE,** | | |
| frozen (Stouffer's) with noodles | 10⅛-oz. meal | 270 |
| **SHRIMP COCKTAIL** canned or | | |
| frozen (Sau-Sea) | 4 oz. | 113 |
| **SHRIMP DINNER,** frozen: | | |
| (Armour) *Classic Lite,* baby | 10½-oz. meal | 260 |
| (Blue Star) *Dining Lite,* creole | 10-oz. meal | 210 |
| (Conagra) *Light & Elegant* | 10-oz. meal | 218 |
| (La Choy) Fresh & Lite, with lobster | | |
| sauce | 10-oz. meal | 240 |

| Food and Description | Measure or Quantity | Calories |
|---|---|---|
| (Stouffer's) *Right Course*, primavera | 9⅝-oz meal | 240 |
| **SLENDER** (Carnation): | | |
| Bar | 1 bar | 135 |
| Dry | 1 packet | 110 |
| Liquid | 10-fl.-oz. can | 220 |
| **SLOPPY HOT DOG SEASONING** | | |
| **MIX** (French's) | 1½-oz. pkg. | 160 |
| **SLOPPY JOE:** | | |
| Canned: | | |
| (Hormel) *Short Orders* | 7½-oz. can | 340 |
| (Libby's): | | |
| Beef | ⅓ cup | 110 |
| Pork | ⅓ cup | 120 |
| Frozen (Banquet) *Cookin' Bag* | 5-oz. pkg. | 199 |
| **SLOPPY JOE SAUCE** | | |
| (Ragú) *Joe Sauce* | 3½ oz. | 50 |
| **SLOPPY JOE SEASONING MIX:** | | |
| *(Durkee) pizza flavor | 1¼ cups | 746 |
| (French's) | 1 pkg. | 128 |
| *(Hunt's) *Manwich* | 5.9-oz. serving | 320 |
| **S'MORES CRUNCH,** cereal (General Mills) | ¾ cup | 120 |
| **SMURF BERRY CRUNCH,** cereal (Post) | 1 cup | 116 |
| **SNACK BAR** (Pepperidge Farm): | | |
| Apple nut, apricot-raspberry or blueberry | 1.7-oz. piece | 170 |
| Brownie nut or date nut | 1½-oz. piece | 190 |
| Chocolate chip or coconut macaroon | 1½-oz. piece | 210 |
| **SNO BALL** (Hostess) | 1 piece | 149 |
| **SOAVE WINE** (Antinori) | 3 fl. oz. | 84 |
| **SOFT DRINK:** | | |
| Sweetened: | | |
| Apple (Slice) | 6 fl. oz. | 98 |
| Birch beer (Canada Dry) | 6 fl. oz. | 82 |
| Bitter lemon: | | |
| (Canada Dry) | 6 fl. oz. | 75 |
| (Schweppes) | 6 fl. oz. | 82 |
| *Bubble Up* | 6 fl. oz. | 73 |
| *Cactus Cooler* (Canada Dry) | 6 fl. oz. | 90 |
| Cherry: | | |
| (Canada Dry) wild | 6 fl. oz. | 98 |
| (Shasta) black | 6 fl. oz. | 81 |
| Cherry-lime (Spree) | 6 fl. oz. | 79 |
| Chocolate (Yoo-Hoo) | 6 fl. oz. | 93 |
| Citrus mist (Shasta) | 6 fl. oz. | 85 |
| Club | Any quantity | 0 |
| Cola: | | |
| *Coca-Cola:* | | |

| Food and Description | Measure or Quantity | Calories |
|---|---|---|
| Regular or caffeine-free | 6 fl. oz. | 71 |
| Classic | 6 fl. oz. | 61 |
| *Jamaica* (Canada Dry) | 6 fl. oz. | 79 |
| *Pepsi-Cola*, regular or *Pepsi Free* | 6 fl. oz. | 80 |
| (Shasta) regular | 6 fl. oz. | 72 |
| (Slice) cherry | 6 fl. oz. | 82 |
| (Spree) | 6 fl. oz. | 73 |
| Collins mix (Canada Dry) | 6 fl. oz. | 60 |
| Cream: | | |
| (Canada Dry) vanilla | 6 fl. oz. | 97 |
| (Schweppes) | 6 fl. oz. | 86 |
| *Dr. Nehi* (Royal Crown) | 6 fl. oz. | 82 |
| *Dr Pepper* | 6 fl. oz. | 75 |
| Fruit punch: | | |
| (Nehi) | 6 fl. oz. | 107 |
| (Shasta) | 6 fl. oz. | 87 |
| Ginger ale: | | |
| (Canada Dry) regular | 6 fl. oz. | 68 |
| (Fanta) | 6 fl. oz. | 60 |
| (Shasta) | 6 fl. oz. | 60 |
| (Spree) | 6 fl. oz. | 60 |
| Ginger beer (Schweppes) | 6 fl. oz. | 70 |
| Grape: | | |
| (Fanta) | 6 fl. oz. | 81 |
| (Hi-C) | 6 fl. oz. | 74 |
| (Nehi) | 6 fl. oz. | 96 |
| (Schweppes) | 6 fl. oz. | 95 |
| Grapefruit (Spree) | 6 fl. oz. | 77 |
| Lemon lime: | | |
| (Minute Maid) | 6 fl.oz. | 67 |
| (Shasta) | 6 fl. oz. | 73 |
| (Spree) | 6 fl. oz. | 77 |
| Lemon-tangerine (Spree) | 6 fl. oz. | 82 |
| *Mello Yello* | 6 fl. oz. | 87 |
| *Mountain Dew* | 6 fl. oz. | 89 |
| *Mr. PiBB* | 6 fl. oz. | 68 |
| Orange: | | |
| (Canada Dry) *Sunrise* | 6 fl. oz. | 97 |
| (Hi-C) | 6 fl. oz. | 74 |
| (Slice) | 6 fl. oz. | 97 |
| Peach (Nehi) | 6 fl. oz. | 102 |
| Quinine or tonic water (Canada Dry; Schweppes) | 6 fl. oz. | 68 |
| Red Pop (Shasta) | 6 fl. oz. | 79 |
| Root beer: | | |
| *Barrelhead* (Canada Dry) | 6 fl. oz. | 82 |
| (Dad's) | 6 fl. oz. | 83 |
| *Rooti* (Canada Dry) | 6 fl. oz. | 82 |

| Food and Description | Measure or Quantity | Calories |
|---|---|---|
| (Shasta) draft | 6 fl. oz. | 77 |
| (Spree) | 6 fl. oz. | 77 |
| *7-Up* | 6 fl. oz. | 72 |
| *Slice* | 6 fl. oz. | 76 |
| *Sprite* | 6 fl. oz. | 68 |
| Strawberry (Shasta) | 6 fl. oz. | 73 |
| Tropical blend (Spree) | 6 fl. oz. | 73 |
| *Upper Ten* (Royal Crown) | 6 fl. oz. | 85 |
| Dietetic: | | |
| Apple (Slice) | 6 fl. oz. | 10 |
| Birch beer (Shasta) | 6 fl. oz. | 2 |
| *Bubble Up* | 6 fl. oz. | 1 |
| Cherry (Shasta) black | 6 fl. oz. | 0 |
| Chocolate (Shasta) | 6 fl. oz. | 0 |
| Coffee (No-Cal) | 6 fl. oz. | 1 |
| Cola: | | |
| (Canada Dry; Shasta) | 6 fl. oz. | 0 |
| *Coca-Cola*, regular or caffeine free | 6 fl. oz. | <1 |
| *Diet Rite* | 6 fl. oz. | <1 |
| *Pepsi*, diet, light or caffeine free | 6 fl. oz. | <1 |
| *RC* | 6 fl. oz. | <1 |
| (Slice) | 6 fl. oz. | 10 |
| Cream (Shasta) | 6 fl. oz. | <1 |
| *Dr Pepper* | 6 fl. oz. | <2 |
| *Fresca* | 6 fl. oz. | 2 |
| Ginger Ale: | | |
| (Canada Dry) | 6 fl. oz. | 1 |
| (Schweppes) | 6 fl. oz. | 2 |
| Grape (Shasta) | 6 fl. oz. | 0 |
| Grapefruit (Shasta) | 6 fl. oz. | 2 |
| Kiwi-passionfruit (Schweppes) mid-calorie royals | 6 fl. oz. | 35 |
| Lemon-lime (*Diet Rite*) | 6 fl.oz. | 2 |
| *Mr. PiBB* | 6 fl. oz. | <1 |
| Orange: | | |
| (Canada Dry; No-Cal) | 6 fl. oz. | 1 |
| (Minute Maid) | 6 fl. oz. | 8 |
| (Shasta) | 6 fl. oz. | <1 |
| Peach, *Diet Rite*, golden | 6 fl. oz. | 1 |
| Peaches 'n cream (Schweppes) mid-calorie royals | 6 fl. oz. | 35 |
| Quinine or tonic (No-Cal) | 6 fl. oz. | 3 |
| Raspberry, *Diet Rite,* red | 6 fl. oz. | 2 |
| *RC 100* (Royal Crown) caffeine free | 6 fl. oz. | <1 |
| *Red Pop (Shasta)* | 6 fl. oz. | 0 |

| Food and Description | Measure or Quantity | Calories |
|---|---|---|
| Root beer: | | |
| *Barrelhead* (Canada Dry) | 6 fl. oz. | 1 |
| (Dad's; Ramblin'; Shasta) | 6 fl. oz. | <1 |
| *7-Up* | 6 fl. oz. | 2 |
| *Slice* | 6 fl. oz. | 13 |
| *Sprite* | 6 fl. oz. | 1 |
| Strawberry-banana (Schweppes) mid-calorie royals | 6 fl. oz. | 35 |
| *Tab,* regular or caffeine free | 6 fl. oz. | <1 |
| **SOLE,** frozen: | | |
| (Frionor) *Norway Gourmet* | 4-oz. fillet | 60 |
| (Mrs. Paul's) fillets, breaded & fried | 6-oz. serving | 280 |
| (Van De Kamp's) batter dipped, french fried | 1 piece | 140 |
| (Weight Watchers) in lemon sauce | 9⅛-oz. meal | 200 |
| **SOUFFLE,** frozen (Stouffer's): | | |
| Corn | 4-oz. serving | 160 |
| Spinach | 4-oz. serving | 140 |
| **SOUP:** | | |
| Canned, regular pack: | | |
| *Asparagus (Campbell), condensed, cream of: | | |
| Regular | 8-oz. serving | 90 |
| *Creamy Natural* | 8-oz. serving | 200 |
| Bean: | | |
| (Campbell): | | |
| *Chunky,* with ham, old fashioned | 11-oz. can | 290 |
| *Condensed, with bacon | 8-oz. serving | 150 |
| (Grandma Brown's) | 8-oz. serving | 182 |
| Bean, black: | | |
| *(Campbell) condensed | 8-oz. serving | 110 |
| (Crosse & Blackwell) | 6½-oz. serving | 80 |
| Beef: | | |
| (Campbell): | | |
| *Chunky:* | | |
| Regular | 10¾-oz. can | 190 |
| Stroganoff | 10¾-oz. can | 300 |
| *Condensed: | | |
| Regular | 8-oz. serving | 80 |
| Broth | 8-oz. serving | 15 |
| Consommé | 8-oz. serving | 25 |
| Noodle, home style | 8-oz. serving | 90 |
| (College Inn) broth | 1 cup | 18 |
| (Swanson) Broth | 7¼-oz. can | 20 |
| *Broccoli (Campbell) condensed, *Creamy Natural* | 8-oz. serving | 140 |

| Food and Description | Measure or Quantity | Calories |
|---|---|---|
| Celery: | | |
| *(Campbell) condensed, | | |
| cream of | 8-oz. serving | 100 |
| *(Rokeach): | | |
| Prepared with milk | 10-oz. serving | 190 |
| Prepared with water | 10-oz. serving | 90 |
| *Cheddar cheese (Campbell) | 8-oz. serving | 130 |
| Chicken: | | |
| (Campbell): | | |
| *Chunky:* | | |
| & rice | 19-oz. can | 280 |
| vegetable | 19-oz. can | 340 |
| *Condensed: | | |
| Alphabet | 8-oz. serving | 80 |
| Broth: | | |
| Plain | 8-oz. serving | 35 |
| & rice | 8-oz. serving | 50 |
| Cream of | 8-oz. serving | 110 |
| Gumbo | 8-oz. serving | 60 |
| Mushroom, creamy | 8-oz. serving | 120 |
| Noodle: | | |
| Regular | 8-oz. serving | 70 |
| *NoodleOs* | 8-oz. serving | 70 |
| & rice | 8-oz. serving | 60 |
| Vegetable | 8-oz. serving | 70 |
| *Semi-condensed, | | |
| *Soup For One,* | | |
| Vegetable, full flavored | 11-oz. serving | 120 |
| (College Inn) broth | 1 cup | 35 |
| (Swanson) broth | 7¼-oz. can | 30 |
| Chili beef (Campbell) *Chunky* | 11-oz. can | 290 |
| Chowder: | | |
| Beef'n vegetable (Hormel) | | |
| *Short Orders* | 7½-oz. can | 120 |
| Clam: | | |
| Manhattan style: | | |
| (Campbell): | | |
| *Chunky* | 19-oz. can | 300 |
| *Condensed | 8-oz. serving | 70 |
| (Crosse & Blackwell) | 6½-oz. serving | 50 |
| *(Snow's) condensed | 7½-oz. serving | 70 |
| New England style: | | |
| *(Campbell): | | |
| Condensed: | | |
| Made with milk | 8-oz. serving | 150 |
| Made with water | 8-oz. serving | 80 |
| Semi-condensed, | | |
| *Soup for One:* | | |
| Made with milk | 11-oz. serving | 190 |

162

| Food and Description | Measure or Quantity | Calories |
|---|---|---|
| Made with water | 11-oz. serving | 130 |
| (Crosse & Blackwell) | 6½-oz. serving | 90 |
| *(Gorton's) | 1 can | 560 |
| *(Snow's) condensed, made with milk | 7½-oz. serving | 140 |
| *Fish (Snow's) condensed, made with milk | 7½-oz. serving | 130 |
| Ham'n potato (Hormel) | 7½-oz. can | 130 |
| Consommé madrilene (Crosse & Blackwell) | 6½-oz. serving | 25 |
| Crab (Crosse & Blackwell) | 6½-oz. serving | 50 |
| Gazpacho (Crosse & Blackwell) | 6½-oz. serving | 30 |
| Ham'n butter bean (Campbell) *Chunky* | 10¾-oz. can | 280 |
| Lentil (Crosse & Blackwell) with ham | 6½-oz. serving | 80 |
| *Meatball alphabet (Campbell) condensed | 8-oz. serving | 100 |
| Minestrone: | | |
| (Campbell): | | |
| *Chunky* | 19-oz. can | 280 |
| *Condensed | 8-oz. serving | 80 |
| (Crosse & Blackwell) | 6½-oz. serving | 90 |
| Mushroom: | | |
| *(Campbell): | | |
| Condensed: | | |
| Cream of | 8-oz. serving | 100 |
| Golden | 8-oz. serving | 80 |
| (Crosse & Blackwell) cream of, bisque | 6½-oz. serving | 90 |
| *(Rokeach) cream of: | | |
| Prepared with milk | 10-oz. serving | 240 |
| Prepared with water | 10-oz. serving | 150 |
| *Noodle (Campbell) & ground beef | 8-oz. serving | 90 |
| *Onion (Campbell): | | |
| Regular | 8-oz. serving | 60 |
| Cream of: | | |
| Made with water | 8-oz. serving | 100 |
| Made with water & milk | 8-oz. serving | 140 |
| *Oyster stew (Campbell): | | |
| Made with milk | 8-oz. serving | 150 |
| Made with water | 8-oz. serving | 80 |
| *Pea, green (Campbell) | 8-oz. serving | 160 |
| Pea, split: | | |
| (Campbell): | | |
| *Chunky,* with ham | 19-oz. can | 400 |
| *Condensed, with ham & bacon | 8-oz. serving | 160 |

| Food and Description | Measure or Quantity | Calories |
|---|---|---|
| (Grandma Brown's) | 8-oz. serving | 184 |
| *Pepper pot (Campbell) | 8-oz. serving | 90 |
| *Potato (Campbell) cream of: | | |
| Regular: | | |
| Made with water | 8-oz. serving | 70 |
| Made with water & milk | 8-oz. serving | 110 |
| *Creamy Natural* | 8-oz. serving | 220 |
| Shav (Gold's) | 8-oz. serving | 25 |
| Shrimp: | | |
| *(Campbell) condensed, cream of: | | |
| Made with milk | 8-oz. serving | 160 |
| Made with water | 8-oz. serving | 90 |
| (Crosse & Blackwell) | 6½-oz. serving | 90 |
| *Spinach (Campbell) condensed, *Creamy Natural* | 8-oz. serving | 160 |
| Steak & potato (Campbell) *Chunky* | 19-oz. can | 340 |
| Tomato: | | |
| (Campbell): | | |
| Condensed: | | |
| Regular: | | |
| Made with milk | 8-oz. serving | 160 |
| Made with water | 8-oz. serving | 90 |
| & rice, old fashioned | 8-oz. serving | 110 |
| *Creamy Natural* | 8-oz. serving | 190 |
| Semi-condensed, *Soup For One,* Royale | 11-oz. serving | 180 |
| *(Rokeach): | | |
| Made with milk | 10-oz. serving | 190 |
| Made with water | 10-oz. serving | 90 |
| Turkey (Campbell) *Chunky* | 18¾-oz. can | 300 |
| Vegetable: | | |
| (Campbell): | | |
| *Chunky:* | | |
| Regular | 19-oz. can | 260 |
| Beef, old fashioned | 19-oz. can | 320 |
| *Condensed: | | |
| Regular | 8-oz. serving | 80 |
| Beef or vegetarian | 10-oz. serving | 70 |
| *Semi-condensed, *Soup For One,* old world | 11-oz. serving | 160 |
| *(Rokeach) vegetarian | 10-oz. serving | 90 |
| Vichyssoise (Crosse & Blackwell) | 6½-oz. serving | 70 |
| *Won ton (Campbell) | 8-oz. serving | 40 |
| Canned, dietetic pack: | | |
| Bean (Pritikin) navy | ½ of 14¾-oz. can | 130 |
| Beef (Campbell) *Chunky,* & mushroom, low sodium | 10¾-oz. can | 210 |

| Food and Description | Measure or Quantity | Calories |
|---|---|---|
| Chicken: | | |
| (Campbell) low sodium: | | |
| Regular, with noodles | 10¾-oz. can | 160 |
| Vegetable | 10¾-oz. can | 240 |
| *(Estee) & vegetable, chunky | 7½-oz. serving | 130 |
| (Pritikin): | | |
| Broth | ½ of 13¾-oz. can | 14 |
| Vegetable | ½ of 14¾-oz. can | 70 |
| Chowder (Pritikin): | | |
| Manhattan | ½ of 14¾-oz. can | 70 |
| New England | ½ of 14¾-oz. can | 118 |
| Lentil (Pritikin) | ½ of 14¾-oz. can | 100 |
| *Minestrone (Estee) | 7½-oz. serving | 165 |
| Mushroom (Campbell) cream of, low sodium | 10½-oz. can | 200 |
| Onion (Campbell) low sodium | 10½-oz. can | 80 |
| Pea, split (Campbell) low sodium | 10¾-oz. can | 240 |
| Tomato: (Campbell) low sodium with tomato pieces | 10½-oz. can | 180 |
| Turkey (Pritikin) vegetable | ½ of 14¾-oz. can | 50 |
| Vegetable (Campbell) *Chunky* low sodium | 10¾-oz. can | 170 |
| Frozen: | | |
| Asparagus (Kettle Ready) cream of | 6 fl. oz. | 62 |
| *Barley & mushroom: | | |
| (Empire Kosher) | 7½-oz. serving | 69 |
| (Tabatchnick) | 8-oz. serving | 92 |
| Bean (Kettle Ready) black | 6 fl. oz. | 154 |
| Bean & barley (Tabatchnick) | 8 oz. | 63 |
| Beef (Kettle Ready) vegetable | 6 fl. oz. | 85 |
| Broccoli, cream of: | | |
| (Kettle Ready) regular | 6 oz. | 95 |
| (Tabatchnick) | 7½ oz. | 90 |
| Cheese, cheddar (Kettle Ready) | 6 oz. | 158 |
| Chicken: | | |
| (Empire Kosher) noodle | 7½-oz. serving | 267 |
| (Kettle Ready): | | |
| Cream of | 6 fl. oz. | 98 |
| Gumbo | 6 fl. oz. | 93 |
| Chowder: | | |
| Clam: | | |
| Boston (Kettle Ready) | 6 oz. | 131 |
| Manhattan: | | |
| (Kettle Ready) | 6 oz. | 69 |
| (Tabatchnick) | 7½ oz. | 94 |
| New England: | | |
| (Kettle Ready) | 6 oz. | 116 |
| (Stouffer's) | 8 oz. | 180 |

| Food and Description | Measure or Quantity | Calories |
|---|---|---|
| (Tabatchnick) | 7½ oz. | 97 |
| Corn & broccoli (Kettle Ready) | 6 oz. | 101 |
| Minestrone (Tabatchnick) | 8 oz. | 147 |
| Mushroom (Kettle Ready) cream of | 6 fl. oz. | 85 |
| Onion (Kettle Ready) | 6 oz. | 42 |
| Pea, split with ham: | | |
| (Kettle Ready) | 6 oz. | 155 |
| (Tabatchnick) | 8 oz. | 186 |
| Potato (Kettle Ready) cream of | 8 oz. | 162 |
| Spinach, cream of: | | |
| (Stouffer's) | 8 oz. | 210 |
| (Tabatchnick) | 7½ oz. | 90 |
| Tomato (Empire Kosher) rice, cream of | 7½ oz. | 227 |
| Vegetable: | | |
| (Empire Kosher) | 7½ oz. | 111 |
| (Kettle Ready) garden | 6 oz. | 85 |
| (Tabatchnick) | 8 oz. | 97 |
| *Won Ton (La Choy) | ½ of 15-oz. pkg. | 50 |
| Mix, regular: | | |
| Beef: | | |
| *Carmel Kosher | 6 fl. oz. | 12 |
| *(Lipton) Cup-A-Soup: | | |
| Noodle | 6 fl. oz. | 45 |
| Lots-A-Noodles | 7 fl. oz. | 120 |
| *(Weight Watchers) broth | 6 fl. oz. | 10 |
| *Chicken: | | |
| Carmel Kosher | 6 fl. oz. | 12 |
| (Lipton): | | |
| Cup-A-Broth | 6 fl. oz. | 25 |
| Cup-A-Soup, & rice | 6 fl. oz. | 45 |
| Country style, hearty | 6 fl. oz. | 73 |
| Lots-A-Noodles, regular | 7 fl. oz. | 120 |
| *Minestrone (Manischewitz) | 6 fl. oz. | 50 |
| *Mushroom: | | |
| Carmel Kosher | 6 fl. oz. | 12 |
| (Lipton): | | |
| Regular, beef | 8 fl. oz. | 40 |
| Cup-A-Soup, cream of | 6 fl. oz. | 82 |
| *Noodle (Lipton): | | |
| With chicken broth | 8 fl. oz. | 70 |
| Giggle Noodle | 8 fl. oz. | 80 |
| *Onion: | | |
| Carmel Kosher | 6 fl. oz. | 12 |
| (Lipton): | | |
| Regular, beef | 8 fl. oz. | 35 |
| Cup-A-Soup | 6 fl. oz. | 30 |
| *Pea, green (Lipton) Cup-A-Soup | 6 fl. oz. | 115 |
| *Pea, split (Manischewitz) | 6 fl. oz. | 45 |

| Food and Description | Measure or Quantity | Calories |
|---|---|---|
| *Tomato (Lipton) *Cup-A-Soup* | 6 fl. oz. | 100 |
| *Tomato onion (Lipton) | 8 fl. oz. | 80 |
| *Vegetable: | | |
| (Lipton): | | |
|   Regular, country | 8 fl. oz. | 80 |
|   *Cup-A-Soup:* | | |
|     Regular, spring | 6 fl. oz. | 41 |
|     Country style, harvest | 6 fl. oz. | 94 |
|     *Lots-A-Noodles,* garden | 7 fl. oz. | 130 |
| (Manischewitz) | 6 fl. oz. | 50 |
| (Southland) frozen | ⅓ of 16-oz. pkg. | 60 |
| *Mix, dietetic: | | |
| (Estee): | | |
|   Beef noodle | 6 fl. oz. | 20 |
|   Chicken noodle | 6 fl. oz. | 25 |
|   Tomato | 6 fl. oz. | 40 |
| (Lipton) *Cup-A-Soup-Trim* | 6 fl. oz. | 10 |
| **SOUP GREENS** (Durkee) | 2⅓-oz. jar | 216 |
| ***SOUTHERN COMFORT:*** | | |
| 80 proof | 1 fl. oz. | 79 |
| 100 proof | 1 fl. oz. | 95 |
| **SOYBEAN CURD OR TOFU** | 2¾" × 1½" × 1" cake | 86 |
| **SOYBEAN OR NUT:** | | |
| Dry roasted (*Soy Ahoy; Soy Town*) | 1 oz. | 139 |
| Oil roasted (*Soy Ahoy; Soy Town*) | | |
|   plain, barbecue or garlic | 1 oz. | 152 |
| **SPAGHETTI:** | | |
| Dry (Pritikin) whole wheat | 1 oz. | 110 |
| Cooked: | | |
|   8-10 minutes, "Al Dente" | 1 cup | 216 |
|   14-20 minutes, tender | 1 cup | 155 |
| Canned: | | |
|   (Franco-American): | | |
|     In meat sauce | 7½-oz. can | 210 |
|     With meatballs in tomato sauce, *SpaghettiOs* | 7⅜-oz. can | 210 |
|     With sliced franks in tomato sauce, *SpaghettiOs* | 7⅜-oz. can | 210 |
|   (Hormel) *Short Orders,* & meatballs in tomato sauce | 7½-oz. can | 210 |
|   (Libby's) & meatballs in tomato sauce | 7½-oz. serving | 189 |
|   Dietetic (Estee) & meatballs | 7½-oz. serving | 240 |
| Frozen: | | |
|   (Banquet) & meat sauce | 8-oz. pkg. | 270 |
|   (Conagra) *Light & Elegant,* & meat sauce | 10¼-oz. entree | 290 |
|   (Morton) & meatball | 10-oz. dinner | 198 |
|   (Stouffer's) *Lean Cuisine* | 11½-oz. pkg. | 280 |

| Food and Description | Measure or Quantity | Calories |
|---|---|---|
| (Weight Watchers) with meat sauce | 10½-oz. meal | 280 |
| **SPAGHETTI SAUCE,** canned: | | |
| Regular pack: | | |
| Garden Style (Ragú) | 4-oz. serving | 80 |
| Marinara: | | |
| (Prince) | 4-oz. serving | 80 |
| (Ragú) | 5-oz. serving | 120 |
| Meat or meat flavored: | | |
| (Hunt's) | 4-oz. serving | 70 |
| (Prego) | 4-oz. serving | 150 |
| (Ragú) regular | 4-oz. serving | 80 |
| Meatless or plain: | | |
| (Prego) | 4-oz. serving | 140 |
| (Ragú) regular | 4-oz. serving | 80 |
| Mushroom: | | |
| (Hain) | 4-oz. serving | 80 |
| (Hunt's) | 4-oz. serving | 70 |
| (Prego Plus) | 4-oz. serving | 130 |
| (Ragú) Extra Thick & Zesty | 4-oz. serving | 110 |
| Sausage & green pepper (Prego Plus) | 4-oz. serving | 170 |
| Veal (Prego Plus) | 4-oz. serving | 150 |
| Dietetic pack: | | |
| (Estee) | 4-oz. serving | 60 |
| (Furman's) low sodium | ½ cup | 83 |
| (Prego) low sodium | ½ cup | 100 |
| (Pritikin) plain or mushroom | 4-oz. serving | 60 |
| **SPAGHETTI SAUCE MIX:** | | |
| *(Durkee) regular | ½ cup | 45 |
| *(French's) with mushrooms | ⅝ cup | 100 |
| (Lawry's) rich & thick | 1½-oz. pkg. | 147 |
| *(Spatini) | ½ cup | 84 |
| *SPAM,* luncheon meat (Hormel): | | |
| Regular, smoke flavored or with cheese chunks | 1-oz. serving | 85 |
| Deviled | 1 T. | 35 |
| **SPARKLING COOLER CITRUS,** *La Croix* (Heileman) | 6 fl. oz. | 107 |
| *SPECIAL K,* cereal (Kellogg's) | 1 cup | 110 |
| **SPINACH:** | | |
| Fresh, whole leaves | ½ cup | 4 |
| Boiled | ½ cup | 18 |
| Canned, regular pack (Allens) solids & liq. | ½ cup | 25 |
| Canned, dietetic pack (Del Monte) No Salt Added | ½ cup | 25 |
| Frozen: | | |

168

| Food and Description | Measure or Quantity | Calories |
|---|---|---|
| (Birds Eye): | | |
| Chopped or leaf | ⅓ pkg. | 28 |
| Creamed | ⅓ pkg. | 60 |
| (Green Giant): | | |
| Creamed | 3.3 oz. | 40 |
| *Harvest Fresh* | 4.5 oz. serving | 25 |
| (McKenzie) chopped or cut | ⅓ pkg. | 25 |
| **SPINACH PUREE,** canned | | |
| (Larsen) low sodium | ½ cup | 22 |
| **SQUASH, SUMMER:** | | |
| Yellow, boiled slices | ½ cup | 13 |
| Zucchini, boiled slices | ½ cup | 9 |
| Canned (Del Monte) zucchini, in tomato sauce | ½ cup | 30 |
| Frozen: | | |
| (Birds Eye) zucchini | ⅓ pkg. | 19 |
| (Larsen) yellow crookneck | 3.3 oz. | 18 |
| (McKenzie) crookneck | ⅓ pkg. | 20 |
| (Mrs. Paul's) sticks, batter dipped, french fried | ⅓ pkg. | 180 |
| **SQUASH, WINTER:** | | |
| Acorn, baked | ½ cup | 56 |
| Hubbard, baked, mashed | ½ cup | 51 |
| Frozen: | | |
| (Birds Eye) | ⅓ pkg. | 43 |
| (Southland) butternut | 4-oz. serving | 45 |
| **STEAK** (See BEEF) | | |
| **STEAK & GREEN PEPPERS,** frozen: | | |
| (Green Giant) | 9-oz. entree | 250 |
| (Swanson) | 8½-oz. entree | 200 |
| **STEAK UMM** | 2 oz. | 180 |
| **STOCK BASE** (French's) beef or chicken | 1 tsp. | 8 |
| **STRAWBERRY:** | | |
| Fresh, capped | ½ cup | 26 |
| Frozen (Birds Eye): | | |
| Halves | ⅓ pkg. | 164 |
| Whole | ¼ pkg. | 89 |
| Whole, quick thaw | ½ pkg. | 125 |
| **STRAWBERRY DRINK** (Hi-C): | | |
| Canned | 6 fl. oz. | 89 |
| *Mix | 6 fl. oz. | 68 |
| **STRAWBERRY FRUIT JUICE,** canned (Smucker's) | 8 fl. oz. | 120 |
| ***STRAWBERRY KRISPIES,*** cereal (Kellogg's) | ¾ cup | 110 |
| **STRAWBERRY NECTAR,** canned (Libby's) | 6 fl. oz. | 60 |

169

| Food and Description | Measure or Quantity | Calories |
|---|---|---|
| **STRAWBERRY PRESERVE** | | |
| **OR JAM:** | | |
| Sweetened: | | |
| (Bama) | 1 T. | 45 |
| (Smucker's) | 1 T. | 53 |
| (Welch's) | 1 T. | 52 |
| Dietetic or low calorie: | | |
| (Estee; Louis Sherry) | 1 T. | 6 |
| (Diet Delight) | 1 T. | 12 |
| (Featherweight) calorie reduced | 1 T. | 16 |
| **STUFFING MIX:** | | |
| *Beef, *Stove Top* | ½ cup | 180 |
| *Chicken: | | |
| *(Bell's) | ½ cup | 224 |
| *(Betty Crocker) | ⅕ pkg. | 180 |
| *Stove Top* | ½ cup | 180 |
| *Cornbread, *Stove Top* | ½ cup | 170 |
| Cube or herb seasoned | | |
| (Pepperidge Farm) | 1 oz. | 110 |
| *Herb (Betty Crocker) | | |
| traditional | ⅙ pkg. | 190 |
| *Pork, *Stove Top* | ½ cup | 170 |
| *Premium Blend (Bell's) | ½ cup | 180 |
| *Ready Mix (Bell's) | ½ cup | 224 |
| White bread (Mrs. Cubbison's) | 1 oz. | 101 |
| **STURGEON,** smoked | 4-oz. serving | 169 |
| **SUCCOTASH:** | | |
| Canned: | | |
| (Comstock) whole kernel | ½ cup | 80 |
| (Larsen) *Freshlike* | ½ cup | 80 |
| (Libby's) cream style | ½ cup | 111 |
| (Stokely-Van Camp) | ½ cup | 85 |
| Frozen: | | |
| (Birds Eye) | ⅓ pkg. | 104 |
| (Frosty Acres) | 3.3 oz. | 100 |
| ***SUDDENLY SALADS** (General | | |
| Mills): | | |
| Macaroni, creamy | ⅙ of pkg. | 200 |
| Pasta, Italian | ⅙ of pkg. | 160 |
| Potato, creamy | ⅙ of pkg. | 250 |
| **SUGAR:** | | |
| Brown | 1 T. | 48 |
| Confectioners' | 1 T. | 30 |
| Granulated | 1 T. | 46 |
| Maple | 1¾″ × 1¼″ × ½″ piece | 104 |
| ***SUGAR CORN POPS**, cereal* | | |
| (Kellogg's) | 1 cup | 110 |
| ***SUGAR CRISP,** cereal (Post)* | ⅞ cup | 112 |

| Food and Description | Measure or Quantity | Calories |
|---|---|---|
| **SUGAR PUFFS,** cereal | | |
| (Malt-O-Meals) | ⅞ cup | 110 |
| **SUGAR SMACKS,** cereal (Kellogg's) | ¾ cup | 110 |
| **SUGAR SUBSTITUTE:** | | |
| (Estee) | 1 tsp. | 12 |
| (Featherweight) | 3 drops | 0 |
| (Pritikin) *Supreme* | 1.76-oz. packet | 3 |
| *Sprinkle Sweet* (Pillsbury) | 1 tsp. | 2 |
| *Sweet'n-it* (Estee) liquid | 5 drops | 0 |
| *Sweet 'N Low:* | | |
| Brown | 1 tsp. | 20 |
| Granulated | 1-gram packet | 4 |
| Liquid | 1 drop | 0 |
| ***SUKIYAKI DINNER** (Chun King) | | |
| stir fry | 6 oz. | 257 |
| **SUNFLOWER SEED** (Fisher): | | |
| In hull, roasted, salted | 1 oz. | 86 |
| Hulled, dry roasted, salted | 1 oz. | 164 |
| Hulled, oil roasted, salted | 1 oz. | 167 |
| **SURIMI** (See CRAB SUBSTITUTE) | | |
| **SUZY Q** (Hostess): | | |
| Banana | 1 piece | 240 |
| Chocolate | 1 piece | 240 |
| **SWEETBREADS,** calf, braised | 4-oz. serving | 191 |
| **SWEET POTATO:** | | |
| Baked, peeled | 5″ × 1″ potato | 155 |
| Canned: | | |
| (Allen's) | 4-oz. serving | 50 |
| (Trappey's) *Sugary Sam:* | | |
| Cut | ½ cup (4.3 oz.) | 110 |
| Whole | ½ cup (4.3 oz.) | 130 |
| Frozen: | | |
| (Mrs. Paul's) candied, with apples | 4-oz. serving | 150 |
| (Stouffer's) & apples | 5-oz. serving | 160 |
| **SWEET & SOUR PORK,** frozen: | | |
| (Chun King) | 13-oz. entree | 394 |
| (La Choy) | 12-oz. entree | 360 |
| **SWISS STEAK,** frozen (Swanson) | 10-oz. dinner | 350 |
| **SWORDFISH,** broiled | 3″ × 3″ × ½″ steak | 218 |
| **SYRUP** (See also TOPPING): | | |
| Regular: | | |
| Apricot (Smucker's) | 1 T. | 50 |
| Blackberry (Smucker's) | 1 T. | 50 |
| Chocolate or chocolate-flavored: | | |
| *Bosco* | 1 T. | 55 |
| (Hershey's) | 1 T. | 40 |
| (Nestlé) *Quik* | 1 oz. | 80 |
| Corn, *Karo,* dark or light | 1 T. | 58 |
| Maple, *Karo,* imitation | 1 T. | 57 |

| Food and Description | Measure or Quantity | Calories |
|---|---|---|
| Pancake or waffle: | | |
| (Aunt Jemima) | 1 T. | 53 |
| *Golden Griddle* | 1 T. | 54 |
| *Karo* | 1 T. | 58 |
| *Log Cabin,* regular or buttered | 1 T. | 56 |
| *Mrs. Butterworth's* | 1 T. | 55 |
| Strawberry (Smucker's) | 1 T. | 50 |
| Dietetic or low calorie: | | |
| Blueberry (Estee) | 1 T. | 4 |
| Chocolate or chocolate-flavored | | |
| (Estee) | 1 T. | 6 |
| Coffee (No-Cal) | 1 T. | 6 |
| Cola (No-Cal) | 1 T. | 0 |
| Maple (S&W) *Nutradiet* | 1 T. | 12 |
| Pancake or waffle: | | |
| (Aunt Jemima) | 1 T. | 29 |
| (Cary's) | 1 T. | 6 |
| (Estee) | 1 T. | 4 |

# T

| Food and Description | Measure or Quantity | Calories |
|---|---|---|
| **TACO:** | | |
| *(Ortega) | 1 oz. | 54 |
| *Mix (Durkee) | ½ cup | 321 |
| Shell (Ortega) | 1 shell | 50 |
| ***TACO BELL RESTAURANTS:*** | | |
| Burrito: | | |
| Bean: | | |
| Green sauce | 6¾-oz. serving | 351 |
| Red sauce | 6¾-oz. serving | 357 |
| Beef: | | |
| Green sauce | 6¾-oz. serving | 398 |
| Red sauce | 6¾-oz. serving | 403 |
| *Supreme:* | | |
| Regular: | | |
| Green sauce | 8½-oz. serving | 407 |
| Red sauce | 8½-oz. serving | 413 |
| Double beef: | | |
| Green sauce | 9-oz. serving | 451 |
| Red sauce | 9-oz. serving | 456 |
| Cinnamon crispas | 1.7-oz. serving | 259 |
| *Enchrito:* | | |
| Green sauce | 7½-oz. serving | 371 |
| Red sauce | 7½-oz. serving | 382 |
| Fajita: | | |
| Chicken | 4¾-oz. serving | 225 |
| Steak | 4¾-oz. serving | 234 |
| Guacamole | ¾-oz. serving | 34 |
| *Meximelt* | 3¾-oz. serving | 266 |
| Nachos: | | |
| Regular | 3¾-oz. serving | 345 |
| *Bellgrande* | 10.1-oz. serving | 648 |
| Pepper, jalapeno | 3½-oz. serving | 20 |
| Pico De Gallo | 1-oz. serving | 8 |
| Pintos & cheese: | | |
| Green sauce | 4½-oz. serving | 184 |
| Red sauce | 4½-oz. serving | 190 |
| Pizza, Mexican | 7.9-oz. serving | 575 |
| Ranch dressing | 2.6-oz. serving | 235 |
| Salsa | .3-oz. serving | 18 |

| Food and Description | Measure or Quantity | Calories |
|---|---|---|
| Sour cream | ¾-oz. serving | 46 |
| Taco: | | |
| Regular | 2¾-oz. serving | 183 |
| *Bellgrande* | 5¾-oz. serving | 355 |
| Light | 6-oz. serving | 410 |
| Soft: | | |
| Regular | 3¼-oz. serving | 338 |
| *Supreme* | 4.4-oz. serving | 275 |
| Super combo | 5-oz. serving | 286 |
| Taco salad: | | |
| With shell | 18.7-oz. serving | 502 |
| With salsa: | | |
| Regular | 21-oz. serving | 941 |
| Without shell | 18.7-oz. serving | 520 |
| Taco sauce: | | |
| Regular | .4-oz. packet | 2 |
| Hot | .4-oz. packet | 2 |
| Tostada: | | |
| Green sauce | 5½-oz. serving | 237 |
| Red sauce | 5½-oz. serving | 243 |
| *TACO JOHN'S:* | | |
| Burrito: | | |
| Bean | 5-oz. serving | 197 |
| Beef | 5-oz. serving | 303 |
| Chicken: | | |
| Regular | 5-oz. serving | 227 |
| With green chili | 12¼-oz. serving | 344 |
| Combo | 5-oz. serving | 250 |
| Smothered: | | |
| With green chili | 12¼-oz. serving | 367 |
| With Texas chili | 12¼-oz. serving | 455 |
| Super: | | |
| Regular | 8¼-oz. serving | 389 |
| With chicken | 8¼-oz. serving | 366 |
| Chimichanga: | | |
| Regular | 12-oz. serving | 464 |
| With chicken | 12-oz. serving | 441 |
| Mexican rice | 8-oz. serving | 340 |
| Nachos: | | |
| Regular | 5-oz. serving | 468 |
| Super | 11¼-oz. serving | 669 |
| *Potato Ole,* large | 6-oz. serving | 414 |
| Taco: | | |
| Regular | 4¼-oz. serving | 178 |
| With chicken | 4¼-oz. serving | 140 |
| Softshell: | | |
| Regular | 5-oz. serving | 224 |
| With chicken | 5-oz. serving | 180 |

| Food and Description | Measure or Quantity | Calories |
|---|---|---|
| Taco Bravo: | | |
| Regular | 6¾-oz. serving | 319 |
| Super | 8-oz. serving | 361 |
| Taco burger | 6-oz. serving | 281 |
| Taco salad: | | |
| Regular: | | |
| Without dressing | 6-oz. serving | 229 |
| With dressing | 8-oz. serving | 359 |
| Chicken: | | |
| Without dressing | 12¼-oz. serving | 377 |
| With dressing | 14¼-oz. serving | 507 |
| Super: | | |
| Without dressing | 12¼-oz. serving | 428 |
| With dressing | 14¼-oz. serving | 558 |
| **TAMALE:** | | |
| Canned: | | |
| (Hormel) beef, *Short Orders* | 7½-oz. can | 270 |
| *Old El Paso,* with chili gravy | 1 tamale | 96 |
| (Pride of Mexico) beef | 1 tamale | 115 |
| Frozen (Hormel) beef | 1 tamale | 130 |
| ***TANG,*** orange, regular | 6 fl. oz. | 87 |
| **TANGERINE OR MANDARIN ORANGE:** | | |
| Fresh (Sunkist) | 1 large tangerine | 39 |
| Canned, solids & liq.: | | |
| Regular pack (Dole) | ½ cup | 76 |
| Dietetic pack: | | |
| (Diet Delight) juice pack | ½ cup | 50 |
| (Featherweight) water pack | ½ cup | 35 |
| (S&W) *Nutradiet* | ½ cup | 28 |
| **TANGERINE DRINK,** canned (Hi-C) | 6 fl. oz. | 90 |
| ***TANGERINE JUICE,*** frozen (Minute Maid) | 6 fl. oz. | 85 |
| **TAPIOCA,** dry, *Minute,* quick cooking | 1 T. | 32 |
| **TAQUITO,** frozen (Van de Kamp's) beef | 8-oz. serving | 490 |
| **TARRAGON** (French's) | 1 tsp. | 5 |
| ***TASTEEOS,*** cereal (Ralston Purina) | 1¼ cups | 110 |
| ***TEA:*** | | |
| Bag: | | |
| (Celestial Seasonings): | | |
| After dinner: | | |
| *Amaretto Nights* or *Swiss Mint* | 1 cup | <3 |
| *Bavarian Chocolate Orange* | 1 cup | 7 |
| Caffeine free | 1 cup | 4 |
| Fruit & tea | 1 cup | <3 |

175

| Food and Description | Measure or Quantity | Calories |
|---|---|---|
| Herb: | | |
|     *Almond Sunset, Cinnamon apple* or *Cranberry Cove* | 1 cup | 3 |
|     *Emperor's Choice* or *Lemon Zinger* | 1 cup | 4 |
|     *Mandarin Orange Spice* or *Orange Zinger* | 1 cup | 5 |
|     *Roastaroma* | 1 cup | 11 |
|     Premium black tea | 1 cup | 3 |
| (Lipton): | | |
|     Plain or flavored | 1 cup | 2 |
|     Herbal: | | |
|       Almond pleasure or cinnamon apple | 1 cup | 2 |
|       Quietly chamomile or toasty spice | 1 cup | 6 |
| (Sahadi) spearmint | 1 cup | 4 |
| Instant (Nestea)100% | 6 fl. oz. | 0 |
| **TEAM,** cereal | 1 cup | 110 |
| **TEA MIX, ICED:** | | |
| *(Lipton) lemon & sugar flavored | 1 cup | 60 |
| *Nestea*, lemon-flavored | 1 cup | 6 |
| *Dietetic, Crystal Light* | 8 fl. oz. | 2 |
| **TEQUILA SUNRISE COCKTAIL,** | | |
| (Mr. Boston) 12½% alcohol | 3 fl. oz. | 120 |
| **TERIYAKI:** | | |
| *Canned (La Choy) chicken | ¾ cup | 85 |
| Frozen: | | |
|     (Chun King) | 13-oz. entree | 379 |
|     (La Choy) Fresh & Light | 10-oz. meal | 240 |
|     (Stouffer's) beef | 9¾-oz. serving | 290 |
| **TERIYAKI BASTE & GLAZE** | | |
| (Kikkoman) | 1 T. | 28 |
| ***TEXTURED VEGETABLE PROTEIN,** | | |
| Morningstar Farms: | | |
|     Breakfast link | 1 link | 73 |
|     Breakfast patties | 1 patty | 100 |
|     Breakfast strips | 1 strip | 37 |
|     *Grillers* | 1 patty | 190 |
| **THURINGER:** | | |
| (Eckrich) *Smoky Tang* | 1-oz. serving | 80 |
| (Hormel): | | |
|     Beefy | 1-oz. serving | 100 |
|     *Old Smokehouse* | 1-oz. serving | 100 |
| (Louis Rich) turkey | 1-oz. serving | 50 |
| (Ohse) beef | 1 oz. | 80 |
| (Oscar Mayer) beef | .8-oz. slice | 69 |
| **TIGER TAILS** (Hostess) | 2¼-oz. piece | 210 |

| Food and Description | Measure or Quantity | Calories |
|---|---|---|
| **TOASTED WHEAT AND RAISINS,** cereal (Nabisco) | 1 oz. | 100 |
| **TOASTER CAKE OR PASTRY:** | | |
| *Pop-Tarts* (Kellogg's): | | |
| Regular: | | |
| Blueberry, brown sugar, cinnamon or cherry | 1 pastry | 210 |
| Strawberry | 1 pastry | 200 |
| Frosted: | | |
| Blueberry, chocolate fudge or strawberry | 1 pastry | 200 |
| Brown sugar cinnamon, cherry, | 1 pastry | 210 |
| Chocolate-vanilla creme | 1 pastry | 220 |
| *Toaster Strudel* (Pillsbury) | 1 slice | 190 |
| *Toastettes* (Nabisco) regular or frosted | 1 piece | 200 |
| *Toast-R-Cake* (Thomas'): | | |
| Blueberry | 1 piece | 108 |
| Bran | 1 piece | 103 |
| Corn | 1 piece | 120 |
| **TOASTIES,** cereal (Post) | 1¼ cups | 107 |
| **TOASTY O'S,** cereal (Malt-O-Meal) | 1¼ cup | 110 |
| **TOFUTTI:** | | |
| Frozen: | | |
| Regular: | | |
| Chocolate supreme or wildberry supreme | 4 fl. oz. | 210 |
| Maple walnut | 4 fl. oz. | 230 |
| Vanilla | 4 fl. oz. | 200 |
| Cuties: | | |
| Chocolate | 1 piece | 140 |
| Vanilla | 1 piece | 130 |
| *Lite Lite* | 4 fl. oz. | 90 |
| Love Drops: | | |
| Cappuccino or chocolate | 4 fl. oz. | 230 |
| Vanilla | 4 fl. oz. | 220 |
| Soft serve: | | |
| Regular | 4 fl. oz. | 158 |
| Hi-Lite: | | |
| Chocolate | 4 fl. oz. | 100 |
| Vanilla | 4 fl. oz. | 90 |
| **TOMATO:** | | |
| Regular, whole | 1 med. tomato | 33 |
| Cherry, whole | 4 pieces | 14 |
| Canned, regular pack, solids & liq.: | | |
| (Contadina) sliced, baby | ½ cup | 50 |
| (Del Monte) stewed | 4 oz. | 37 |

| Food and Description | Measure or Quantity | Calories |
|---|---|---|
| (Hunt's): | | |
|    Crushed | ½ cup | 25 |
|    Stewed | ½ cup (4 oz.) | 35 |
|    Whole | 4 oz. | 20 |
| (La Victoria) green, whole | 1 oz. | 8 |
| Canned, dietetic pack, solids & liq.: | | |
|    (Del Monte) No Salt Added | ½ cup | 35 |
|    (Featherweight) | ½ cup | 20 |
|    (Furman's) low sodium | ½ cup | 72 |
|    (Hunt's) whole | 4 oz. | 20 |
| **TOMATO & PEPPER, HOT CHILI,** *Old El Paso,* Jalapeño | ¼ cup | 13 |
| **TOMATO JUICE, CANNED:** | | |
| Regular pack: | | |
|    (Ardmore Farms) | 6-fl.-oz. can | 36 |
|    (Campbell; Libby's) | 6-fl.-oz. can | 35 |
|    (Hunt's) | 6 fl. oz. | 30 |
|    (Musselman's) | 6-fl.-oz. can | 30 |
| Dietetic pack (Diet Delight; Featherweight) | 6 fl. oz. | 35 |
| **TOMATO JUICE COCKTAIL,** canned: | | |
| (Ocean Spray) *Firehouse Jubilee* | 6 fl. oz. | 44 |
| *SnapE-Tom* | 6 fl. oz. | 40 |
| **TOMATO PASTE,** canned: | | |
| Regular pack: | | |
|    (Contadina) Italian | 6-oz. serving | 210 |
|    (Del Monte) | 6-oz. can | 150 |
|    (Hunt's) Italian style | 6 oz. | 150 |
| Dietetic (Featherweight) low sodium | 6-oz. can | 150 |
| **TOMATO, PICKLED** (Claussen) green | 1 piece | 6 |
| **TOMATO PUREE,** canned: | | |
| Regular (Contadina) heavy | 1 cup | 100 |
| Dietetic (Featherweight) | 1 cup | 90 |
| **TOMATO SAUCE,** canned: | | |
| (Contadina) regular | 1 cup | 90 |
| (Del Monte): | | |
|    Regular or No Salt Added | 1 cup | 70 |
|    Hot | ½ cup | 40 |
|    With tomato bits | 1 cup | 92 |
|    (Furman's) | ½ cup | 58 |
| (Hunt's): | | |
|    Regular or with bits | 4 oz. | 30 |
|    With cheese | 4 oz. | 45 |
|    Herbs | 4 oz. | 80 |
| **TOM COLLINS** (Mr. Boston) 12½% alcohol | 3 fl. oz. | 111 |
| ***TOM COLLINS MIX,** | | |

| Food and Description | Measure or Quantity | Calories |
|---|---|---|
| (Bar-Tender's) | 6 fl. oz. | 177 |
| **TONGUE,** beef, braised | 4-oz. serving | 277 |
| **TOPPING:** | | |
| Regular: | | |
| Butterscotch (Smucker's) | 1 T. | 70 |
| Caramel (Smucker's) regular | 1 T. | 70 |
| Chocolate fudge (Hershey's) | 1 T. | 50 |
| Nut (Planters) | 1 oz. | 180 |
| Pecans in syrup (Smucker's) | 1 T. | 65 |
| Pineapple (Smucker's) | 1 T. | 65 |
| Strawberry (Smucker's) | 1 T. | 60 |
| Walnuts in syrup (Smucker's) | 1 T. | 65 |
| Dietetic, chocolate (Diet Delight) | 1 T. | 16 |
| **TOPPING, WHIPPED:** | | |
| Regular: | | |
| *Cool Whip* (Birds Eye) dairy | 1 T. | 16 |
| (Johanna) aerosol | 1 T. | 8 |
| *Lucky Whip,* aerosol | 1 T. | 12 |
| Dietetic (Featherweight) | 1 T. | 3 |
| *Mix: | | |
| Regular, *Dream Whip* | 1 T. | 5 |
| Dietetic (D-Zerta; Estee) | 1 T. | 4 |
| *TOP RAMEN,* beef (Nissin Foods) | 3-oz. serving | 390 |
| **TORTELLINI,** frozen: | | |
| (Armour) *Classics Lite,* with meat | 10-oz. dinner | 250 |
| (Buitoni): | | |
| Cheese filled, verdi | 2.6-oz. serving | 220 |
| Meat filled | 2.5-oz. entree | 223 |
| (Stouffer's): | | |
| Cheese filled, with tomato sauce | 9⅝-oz. meal | 360 |
| Veal stuffed, in Alfredo sauce | 8⅝-oz. meal | 500 |
| **TORTILLA** (Amigos) | 6″ × ⅛″ tortilla | 111 |
| **TOSTADA,** frozen (Van de Kamp's) | 8½-oz. serving | 530 |
| **TOSTADA SHELL** (*Old El Paso*) | 1 shell | 57 |
| *TOTAL,* cereal | 1 cup | 110 |
| **TRIPE,** canned (Libby's) | 6-oz. serving | 290 |
| **TRIPLE SEC LIQUEUR** | | |
| (Mr. Boston) | 1 fl. oz. | 79 |
| *TRIX,* cereal (General Mills) | 1 cup | 110 |
| **TUNA:** | | |
| Canned in oil: | | |
| (Bumble Bee): | | |
| Chunk, light, solids & liq. | ½ cup | 265 |
| Solid, white, solids & liq. | ½ cup | 285 |
| (Carnation) solids & liq. | 6½-oz. can | 427 |
| Canned in water: | | |
| (Breast O'Chicken) | 6½-oz. can | 211 |
| (Bumble Bee): | | |
| Chunk, light, solids & liq. | ½ cup | 117 |

| Food and Description | Measure or Quantity | Calories |
|---|---|---|
| Solid, white, solids & liq. | ½ cup | 126 |
| (Featherweight) light, chunk | 6½-oz. can | 210 |
| *TUNA HELPER* (General Mills): | | |
| Au gratin | ⅕ of pkg. | 300 |
| Cold salad | ⅕ of pkg. | 440 |
| Country dumplings or noodles cheese | ⅕ pkg. | 230 |
| Creamy noodle | ⅕ pkg. | 280 |
| Tuna tetrazzini | ⅕ of pkg. | 270 |
| **TUNA NOODLE CASSEROLE,** frozen (Stouffer's) | 10-oz. meal | 310 |
| **TUNA PIE,** frozen: | | |
| (Banquet) | 8-oz. pie | 395 |
| (Morton) | 8-oz. pie | 370 |
| **TUNA SALAD:** | | |
| Home recipe | 4-oz. serving | 193 |
| Canned (Carnation) | ¼ of 7½-oz. can | 100 |
| **TURF & SURF DINNER,** frozen (Armour) *Classic Lights* | 10-oz. meal | 250 |
| **TURKEY:** | | |
| Barbecued (Louis Rich) breast, half | 1 oz. | 40 |
| Packaged: | | |
| (Carl Buddig): | | |
| Regular | 1 oz. | 50 |
| Ham or salami | 1 oz. | 40 |
| *Hebrew National,* breast | 1 oz. | 37 |
| (Hormel) breast | 1 slice | 30 |
| (Louis Rich): | | |
| Turkey bologna | 1-oz. slice | 60 |
| Turkey cotto salami | 1-oz. slice | 50 |
| Turkey ham, chopped | 1-oz. slice | 45 |
| Turkey pastrami | 1-oz. slice | 35 |
| (Ohse): | | |
| Oven cooked | 1 oz. | 30 |
| Turkey bologna | 1 oz. | 70 |
| Turkey salami | 1 oz. | 50 |
| (Oscar Mayer) breast, oven roasted | .7-oz. slice | 23 |
| Roasted: | | |
| Flesh & skin | 4-oz. serving | 253 |
| Dark meat | 2½″ × 1⅝″ × ¼″ slice | 43 |
| Light meat | 4″ × 2″ × ¼″ slice | 75 |
| Smoked (Louis Rich): | | |
| Drumsticks | 1 oz. (without bone) | 40 |
| Wing drumettes | 1 oz. (without bone) | 45 |
| **TURKEY DINNER OR ENTREE,** frozen: | | |
| (Banquet): | | |
| American Favorites | 11-oz. dinner | 320 |
| Extra Helping | 9-oz. dinner | 723 |

| Food and Description | Measure or Quantity | Calories |
|---|---|---|
| (Conagra) *Light & Elegant,* sliced | 8-oz. entree | 230 |
| (Morton) | 10-oz. dinner | 226 |
| (Stouffer's): | | |
| Regular, tetrazzini | 10-oz. meal | 380 |
| *Lean Cuisine,* Dijon | 9½-oz. meal | 270 |
| *Right Course,* sliced, in curry sauce with rice pilaf | 8¾-oz. meal | 320 |
| (Swanson): | | |
| Regular | 8¾-oz. entree | 250 |
| *Hungry Man* | 18½-oz. dinner | 590 |
| (Weight Watchers) stuffed, breast | 8½-oz. meal | 260 |
| **TURKEY NUGGET,** frozen (Empire Kosher) | ¼ of 12-oz. pkg. | 255 |
| **TURKEY PATTY,** frozen (Empire Kosher) | ¼ of 12-oz. pkg. | 188 |
| **TURKEY PIE,** frozen: | | |
| (Banquet): | | |
| Regular | 8-oz. pie | 526 |
| Supreme | 8-oz. pie | 430 |
| (Empire Kosher) | 8-oz. pie | 491 |
| (Morton) | 7-oz. pie | 420 |
| (Stouffer's) | 10-oz. pie | 540 |
| (Swanson) chunky | 10-oz. pie | 530 |
| **TURKEY TETRAZZINI,** frozen: | | |
| (Stouffer's) | 6-oz. serving | 240 |
| (Weight Watchers) | 10-oz. pkg. | 310 |
| **TURNIP GREENS,** canned | | |
| (Allen's) chopped, solids & liq. | ½ cup | 20 |
| **TURNIP ROOTS,** frozen | | |
| (McKenzie) diced | 1 oz. | 4 |
| **TURNOVER:** | | |
| Frozen (Pepperidge Farm): | | |
| Apple or cherry | 1 turnover | 310 |
| Blueberry, peach or raspberry | 1 turnover | 320 |
| Refrigerated (Pillsbury) | 1 turnover | 170 |
| *TWINKIE* (Hostess) | 1 piece | 160 |

# U

| Food and Description | Measure or Quantity | Calories |
|---|---|---|
| **UFO'S,** canned (Franco-American): | | |
| Regular | 7½ oz. | 180 |
| With meteors | 7½ oz. | 240 |

# V

| Food and Description | Measure or Quantity | Calories |
|---|---|---|
| **VALPOLICELLA WINE** (Antinori) | 3 fl. oz. | 84 |
| *VANDERMINT,* liqueur | 1 fl. oz. | 90 |
| **VANILLA EXTRACT** | | |
| (Virginia Dare) | 1 tsp. | 10 |
| **VEAL,** broiled, medium cooked: | | |
| Loin chop | 4 oz. | 265 |
| Rib, roasted | 4 oz. | 305 |
| Steak or cutlet, lean & fat | 4 oz. | 245 |
| **VEAL DINNER,** frozen: | | |
| (Armour) *Dinner Classics,* | | |
| parmigiana | 10¾-oz. meal | 400 |
| (Morton) parmigiana | 10-oz. dinner | 252 |
| (Swanson) parmigiana, | | |
| *Hungry Man* | 20-oz. dinner | 640 |
| (Weight Watchers) parmigiana, | | |
| 2-compartment | 8.625-oz. meal | 230 |
| **VEAL STEAK,** frozen (Hormel): | | |
| Regular | 4-oz. serving | 130 |
| Breaded | 4-oz. serving | 240 |
| **VEGETABLE BOUILLON** | | |
| (Herb-Ox): | | |
| Cube | 1 cube | 6 |
| Packet | 1 packet | 12 |
| **VEGETABLE JUICE COCKTAIL:** | | |
| Regular, *V-8* | 6 fl. oz. | 35 |
| Dietetic: | | |
| (S&W) *Nutradiet,* low sodium | 6 fl. oz. | 35 |
| *V-8,* low sodium | 6 fl. oz. | 40 |
| **VEGETABLES IN PASTRY,** | | |
| frozen (Pepperidge Farm): | | |
| Asparagus with mornay sauce or | | |
| broccoli with cheese | 3¾ oz. | 250 |
| Cauliflower & cheese sauce | 3¾ oz. | 220 |
| Spinach almondine | 3¾ oz. | 260 |
| Zucchini provencal | 3¾ oz. | 210 |
| **VEGETABLES, MIXED:** | | |
| Canned, regular pack: | | |
| (Del Monte) solids & liq. | ½ cup | 40 |

| Food and Description | Measure or Quantity | Calories |
|---|---|---|
| (La Choy) drained: | | |
| Chinese | ⅓ of 14-oz. pkg. | 12 |
| Chop Suey | ½ cup | 9 |
| (Veg-All) | ½ cup | 35 |
| Canned, dietetic pack: | | |
| (Featherweight) | ½ cup | 40 |
| (Larsen) *Fresh-Lite* | ½ cup | 35 |
| Frozen: | | |
| (Birds Eye): | | |
| Regular: | | |
| Broccoli, cauliflower & carrots in cheese sauce | 5 oz. | 100 |
| Carrots, peas & onions, deluxe | ⅓ pkg. | 52 |
| Medley, in butter sauce | ⅓ of 10-oz. pkg. | 62 |
| *Farm Fresh:* | | |
| Broccoli, cauliflower & carrot strips | 3.2 oz. | 25 |
| Brussels sprouts, cauliflower & carrots | 3.2 oz. | 30 |
| *Stir Fry,* Chinese style | ⅓ pkg. | 35 |
| (Chun King) chow mein, drained | 4 oz. | 32 |
| (Frosty Acres): | | |
| Regular | 3.3 oz. | 65 |
| Dutch | 3.2 oz. | 30 |
| Oriental | 3.2 oz. | 25 |
| Soup mix | 3 oz. | 45 |
| Stew | 3 oz. | 42 |
| Swiss mix | 3 oz. | 25 |
| (Green Giant): | | |
| Regular: | | |
| Broccoli, cauliflower & carrots in cheese sauce | ½ cup | 60 |
| Corn, broccoli bounty | ½ cup | 60 |
| *Harvest Fresh* | ½ cup | 60 |
| *Harvest Get Togethers:* | | |
| Broccoli-cauliflower medley | ½ cup | 60 |
| Broccoli fanfare | ½ cup | 80 |
| (La Choy) stir fry | 4 oz. | 40 |
| (Larsen): | | |
| Regular or chuckwagon blend | 3.3 oz. | 70 |
| California blend or Italian blend | 3.3 oz. | 30 |
| Oriental blend | 3.3 oz. | 25 |
| (Southland): | | |
| Gumbo | ⅕ of 16-oz. pkg. | 40 |
| Stew | 4 oz. | 60 |
| **VEGETABLE STEW,** canned *Dinty Moore* (Hormel) | 7½-oz. serving | 170 |

| Food and Description | Measure or Quantity | Calories |
|---|---|---|
| **"VEGETARIAN FOODS":** | | |
| Canned or dry: | | |
| Chicken, fried (Loma Linda) with gravy | 1½-oz. piece | 70 |
| Chili (Worthington) | ½ cup | 177 |
| Choplet (Worthington) | 1 choplet | 50 |
| Dinner cuts (Loma Linda) drained | 1 piece | 60 |
| Dinner loaf (Loma Linda) | ¼ cup | 50 |
| Franks, big (Loma Linda) | 1.9-oz. frank | 100 |
| Franks, sizzle (Loma Linda) | 2.2-oz. frank | 85 |
| *FriChik* (Worthington) | 1 piece | 75 |
| Little links (Loma Linda) drained | .8-oz. link | 40 |
| Non-meatballs (Worthington) | 1 meatball | 32 |
| Nuteena (Loma Linda) | ½" slice | 160 |
| Patty mix (Loma Linda) | ¼ cup | 50 |
| *Prime Stakes* | 1 slice | 171 |
| Proteena (Loma Linda) | ½" slice | 140 |
| Sandwich spread (Loma Linda) | 1 T. | 23 |
| *Soyagen, all purpose powder (Loma Linda) | 1 cup | 130 |
| Soyameat (Worthington): | | |
| Beef, sliced | 1 slice | 44 |
| Chicken, diced | 1 oz. | 40 |
| Soyameal, any kind (Worthington) | 1 oz. | 120 |
| Stew pack (Loma Linda) drained | 2 oz. | 70 |
| Super links (Worthington) | 1 link | 110 |
| Swiss steak with gravy (Loma Linda) | 1 steak | 140 |
| Vegelona (Loma Linda) | ½" slice | 100 |
| Vega-links (Worthington) | 1 link | 55 |
| Wheat protein | 4 oz. | 124 |
| *Worthington 209* | 1 slice | 58 |
| Frozen: | | |
| Beef pie (Worthington) | 1 pie | 278 |
| Bologna (Loma Linda) | 1 oz. | 75 |
| Chicken, fried (Loma Linda) | 2-oz. serving | 180 |
| *Chic-Ketts* (Worthington) | 1 oz. | 53 |
| Corned beef, sliced (Worthington) | 1 slice | 32 |
| *Fri Pats* (Worthington) | 1 patty | 204 |
| Meatballs (Loma Linda) | 1 meatball | 63 |
| Meatless salami (Worthington) | 1 slice | 44 |
| *Prosage* (Worthington) | 1 link | 60 |
| Smoked beef, slices (Worthington) | 1 slice | 14 |
| *Wham*, roll (Worthington) | 1 slice | 36 |

185

| Food and Description | Measure or Quantity | Calories |
|---|---|---|
| **VERMOUTH:** | | |
| Dry & extra dry (Lejon; Noilly Pratt) | 1 fl. oz. | 33 |
| Sweet (Lejon; Taylor) | 1 fl. oz. | 45 |
| **VICHY WATER** (Schweppes) | Any quantity | 0 |
| **VINEGAR** | 1 T. | 2 |

# W

| Food and Description | Measure or Quantity | Calories |
|---|---|---|
| **WAFFELOS**, cereal (Ralston Purina) | 1 cup | 110 |
| **WAFFLE**, frozen: | | |
| (Aunt Jemima) jumbo | 1 waffle | 86 |
| (Eggo): | | |
| Apple cinnamon | 1 waffle | 150 |
| Blueberry or strawberry | 1 waffle | 130 |
| Home style | 1 waffle | 120 |
| **WALNUT**, English or Persian (Diamond A) | 1 cup | 679 |
| **WALNUT FLAVORING**, black (Durkee) imitation | 1 tsp. | 4 |
| **WATER CHESTNUT**, canned: | | |
| (Chun King) whole, drained | ½ of 8½-oz. can | 85 |
| (La Choy) drained | ¼ cup | 16 |
| **WATERCRESS**, trimmed | ½ cup | 3 |
| **WATERMELON:** | | |
| Wedge | 4″ × 8″ wedge | 111 |
| Diced | ½ cup | 21 |
| **WELSH RAREBIT:** | | |
| Home recipe | 1 cup | 415 |
| Frozen: | | |
| (Green Giant) | 5-oz. serving | 219 |
| (Stouffer's) | 5-oz. serving | 350 |
| **WENDY'S** | | |
| Bacon, breakfast | 1 strip | 55 |
| Bacon cheeseburger on white bun | 1 burger | 460 |
| Breakfast sandwich | 1 sandwich | 370 |
| Buns: | | |
| Wheat, multi-grain | 1 bun | 135 |
| White | 1 bun | 160 |
| Chicken sandwich on multi-grain bun | 1 sandwich | 320 |
| Chili: | | |
| Regular | 8 oz. | 260 |
| Large | 12 oz. | 390 |
| Condiments: | | |
| Bacon | ½ strip | 30 |
| Cheese, American | 1 slice | 70 |
| Onion rings | .3-oz. piece | 4 |
| Pickle, dill | 4 slices | 1 |

| Food and Description | Measure or Quantity | Calories |
|---|---|---|
| Relish | .3-oz. serving | 14 |
| Tomato | 1 slice | 2 |
| Danish | 1 piece | 360 |
| Drinks: | | |
| Coffee | 6 fl. oz. | 2 |
| Cola: | | |
| Regular | 12 fl. oz | 110 |
| Dietetic | 12 fl. oz. | Tr. |
| Fruit flavored drink | 12 fl. oz. | 110 |
| Hot chocolate | 6 fl. oz. | 100 |
| Milk: | | |
| Regular | 8 fl. oz. | 150 |
| Chocolate | 8 fl. oz. | 210 |
| Non-cola | 12 fl. oz. | 100 |
| Orange juice | 6 fl. oz. | 80 |
| Egg, scrambled | 1 order | 190 |
| Frosty dairy dessert: | | |
| Small | 12 fl. oz. | 400 |
| Medium | 16 fl. oz. | 533 |
| Large | 20 fl. oz. | 667 |
| Hamburger: | | |
| Double, on white bun | 1 burger | 560 |
| Kids Meal | 1 burger | 220 |
| Single: | | |
| On wheat bun | 1 burger | 340 |
| On white bun | 1 burger | 350 |
| Omelet: | | |
| Ham & cheese | 1 omelet | 250 |
| Ham, cheese & mushroom | 1 omelet | 290 |
| Mushroom, onion & green pepper | 1 omelet | 210 |
| Potato: | | |
| Baked, hot stuffed: | | |
| Plain | 1 potato | 250 |
| Broccoli & cheese | 1 potato | 500 |
| Cheese | 1 potato | 590 |
| Chicken à la King | 1 potato | 350 |
| Sour cream & chives | 1 potato | 460 |
| Stroganoff & sour cream | 1 potato | 490 |
| French fries | regular order | 280 |
| Home fries | 1 order | 360 |
| Salad Bar, *Garden Spot*: | | |
| Alfalfa sprouts | 2 oz. | 20 |
| Bacon bits | ⅛ oz. | 10 |
| Blueberries, fresh | 1 T. | 8 |
| Breadstick | 1 piece | 20 |
| Broccoli | ½ cup | 14 |
| Cantaloupe | 1 piece (2 oz.) | 4 |
| Carrot | ¼ cup | 12 |
| Cauliflower | ½ cup | 14 |

| Food and Description | Measure or Quantity | Calories |
|---|---|---|
| Cheese: | | |
| American, imitation | 1 oz. | 70 |
| Cheddar, imitation | 1 oz. | 90 |
| Cottage | ½ cup | 110 |
| Mozzarella, imitation | 1 oz. | 90 |
| Swiss, imitation | 1 oz. | 80 |
| Chow mein noodles | ¼ cup | 60 |
| Coleslaw | ½ cup | 90 |
| Crouton | 1 piece | 2 |
| Cucumber | ¼ cup | 4 |
| Mushroom | ¼ cup | 6 |
| Onions, red | 1 T. | 4 |
| Orange, fresh | 1 piece | 5 |
| Pasta salad | ½ cup | 134 |
| Peas, green | ½ cup | 60 |
| Peaches, in syrup | 1 piece | 8 |
| Peppers: | | |
| Banana or mild pepperoncini | 1 T. | 18 |
| Bell | ¼ cup | 4 |
| Jalapeño | 1 T. | 9 |
| Pineapple chunks in juice | ½ cup | 80 |
| Tomato | 1 oz. | 6 |
| Turkey ham | ¼ cup | 46 |
| Watermelon, fresh | 1 piece (1 oz.) | 1 |
| Salad dressing: | | |
| Regular: | | |
| Blue cheese | 1 T. | 60 |
| French, red | 1 T. | 70 |
| Italian, golden | 1 T. | 45 |
| Oil | 1 T. | 130 |
| Ranch | 1 T. | 80 |
| Thousand Island | 1 T. | 70 |
| Dietetic: | | |
| Bacon & tomato | 1 T. | 45 |
| Cucumber, creamy | 1 T. | 50 |
| Italian | 1 T. | 25 |
| Thousand Island | 1 T. | 45 |
| Wine vinegar | 1 T. | 2 |
| Salad, Side, pick-up window | 1 salad | 110 |
| Salad, taco | 1 salad | 390 |
| Sausage | 1 patty | 200 |
| Toast: | | |
| Regular, with margarine | 1 slice | 125 |
| French | 1 slice | 200 |
| WESTERN DINNER, frozen: | | |
| (Banquet) American Favorites | 11-oz. dinner | 513 |
| (Morton) regular | 10-oz. dinner | 289 |
| (Swanson) *Hungry Man* | 17½-oz. dinner | 750 |
| *WHEATENA,* cereal | ¼ cup | 112 |

| Food and Description | Measure or Quantity | Calories |
|---|---|---|
| **WHEAT FLAKES CEREAL** | | |
| (Featherweight) | 1¼ cups | 100 |
| **WHEAT GERM CEREAL** | | |
| (Kretschmer) | ¼ cup | 110 |
| **WHEAT GERM, RAW** (Elam's) | 1 T. | 28 |
| ***WHEAT HEARTS,*** cereal | | |
| (General Mills) | 1 oz. | 110 |
| ***WHEATIES,*** cereal | 1 cup | 110 |
| **WHEAT & OATMEAL CEREAL,** | | |
| hot (Elam's) | 1 oz. | 105 |
| **WHISKEY SOUR COCKTAIL** | | |
| (Mr. Boston) | 3 fl. oz. | 120 |
| **\*WHISKEY SOUR MIX** | | |
| (Bar-Tender's) | 3½ fl. oz. | 177 |
| ***WHITE CASTLE:*** | | |
| Bun only | .9-oz. bun | 74 |
| Cheese only | 1 piece | 31 |
| Cheeseburger | 1 sandwich | 200 |
| Chicken sandwich | 1 sandwich | 186 |
| Fish sandwich | 1 sandwich | 155 |
| French fries | 1 order | 301 |
| Hamburger | 1 sandwich | 161 |
| Onion chips | 1 order | 329 |
| Onion rings | 1 order | 245 |
| Sausage & egg sandwich | 1 sandwich | 322 |
| Sausage sandwich | 1 sandwich | 196 |
| **WHITEFISH, LAKE:** | | |
| Baked, stuffed | 4 oz. | 244 |
| Smoked | 4 oz. | 176 |
| ***WIENER WRAP*** (Pillsbury) | 1 piece | 60 |
| **WILD BERRY DRINK,** | | |
| canned (Hi-C) | 6 fl. oz. | 88 |
| ***WINCHELL'S DONUT HOUSE:*** | | |
| Buttermilk, old fashioned | 2-oz. piece | 249 |
| Cake, devil's food, iced | 2-oz. piece | 241 |
| Cinnamon crumb | 2-oz. piece | 240 |
| Iced, chocolate | 2-oz. piece | 227 |
| Raised, glazed | 1¾-oz. piece | 212 |
| **WINE** (See specific type, such as CHIANTI, SHERRY, etc.) | | |
| **WINE, COOKING** (Regina): | | |
| Burgundy or sauterne | ¼ cup | 2 |
| Sherry | ¼ cup | 20 |
| **WINE COOLER** (Bartles & Jaymes): | | |
| Original white | 6 oz. | 92 |
| Premium berry | 6 oz. | 92 |
| Premium red | 6 oz. | 97 |

# Y

| Food and Description | Measure or Quantity | Calories |
|---|---|---|
| **YEAST, BAKER'S** (Fleischmann's): | | |
| Dry, active | 1 packet | 20 |
| Fresh & household, active | .6-oz. cake | 15 |
| **YOGURT:** | | |
| Regular: | | |
| Plain: | | |
| (Dannon): | | |
| Low-fat | 8-oz. cont. | 110 |
| Non-fat | 8-oz. cont. | 140 |
| (Friendship) | 8-oz. container | 170 |
| (Johanna) | 8-oz. container | 150 |
| *Lite-Line* (Borden) | 8-oz. container | 140 |
| (Meadow Gold) | 8-oz. container | 160 |
| (Whitney's) | 6-oz. container | 150 |
| *Yoplait* | 6-oz. container | 130 |
| Apple: | | |
| (Dannon) dutch, Fruit-on-the-Bottom | 8-oz. container | 240 |
| *Yoplait* | 6-oz. container | 190 |
| Apple-cinnamon, *Yoplait, Breakfast Yogurt* | 6-oz. container | 220 |
| Apple & raisins (Whitney's) | 6-oz. container | 200 |
| Apricot (Bison) | 8-oz. container | 262 |
| Banana: | | |
| (Dannon) Fruit-on-the-bottom | 8-oz. container | 240 |
| *Yoplait* | 6-oz. container | 190 |
| Blueberry: | | |
| (Breyer's) | 8-oz. container | 260 |
| (Dannon) *Fresh Flavors* | 8-oz. container | 200 |
| (Mountain High) | 8-oz. container | 220 |
| (Sweet'N Low) | 8-oz. container | 150 |
| (Whitney's) | 6-oz. container | 200 |
| *Yoplait*, custard style | 6-oz. container | 190 |
| Boysenberry: | | |
| (Dannon) Fruit-on-the-Bottom | 8-oz. container | 240 |
| (Sweet'N Low) | 8-oz. container | 150 |
| Cherry: | | |
| (Breyer's) black | 8-oz. container | 270 |

| Food and Description | Measure or Quantity | Calories |
|---|---|---|
| (Dannon) Fruit-on-the-Bottom | 8-oz. container | 240 |
| (Sweet 'n Low) | 8-oz. container | 150 |
| (Whitney's) | 6-oz. container | 200 |
| *Yoplait, Breakfast Yogurt,* with almonds | 6-oz. container | 210 |
| Cherry-vanilla (Borden) *Lite Line* | 8-oz. container | 240 |
| Coffee: | | |
| (Colombo; Dannon) | 8-oz. container | 200 |
| (Johanna) | 8-oz. container | 220 |
| Exotic fruit (Dannon) Fruit-on-the-Bottom | 8-oz. container | 240 |
| Lemon: | | |
| (Dannon) *Fresh Flavors* | 8-oz. container | 200 |
| (Johanna) | 8-oz.container | 220 |
| (Sweet'N Low) | 8-oz. container | 150 |
| (Whitney's) | 6-oz. container | 200 |
| *Yoplait:* | | |
| Regular | 6-oz. container | 190 |
| *Custard Style* | 6-oz. container | 190 |
| Mixed berries (Dannon): | | |
| Extra Smooth | 4.4-oz. container | 130 |
| Fruit-on-the-Bottom | 8-oz. container | 240 |
| Orange, *Yoplait,* custard style | 6-oz. container | 190 |
| Orange supreme (New Country) | 8-oz. container | 210 |
| Orchard, *Yoplait, Breakfast Yogurt* | 6-oz. container | 240 |
| Peach: | | |
| (Breyer's) | 8-oz. container | 270 |
| (Dannon) Fruit-on-the-Bottom | 8-oz. container | 240 |
| (Friendship) | 8-oz. container | 240 |
| *Lite-Line* (Borden) | 8-oz. container | 230 |
| (Sweet'N Low) | 8-oz. container | 150 |
| (Whitney's) | 6-oz. container | 200 |
| Peach melba (Colombo) | 8-oz. container | 230 |
| Piña colada: | | |
| (Dannon) Fruit-on-the-Bottom | 8-oz. container | 240 |
| (Friendship) | 8-oz. container | 230 |
| *Yoplait,* custard style | 6-oz. container | 190 |
| Pineapple: | | |
| (Breyer's) | 8-oz. container | 270 |
| (Light n' Lively) | 8-oz. container | 240 |
| *Yoplait,* custard style | 6-oz. container | 190 |
| Raspberry: | | |
| (Breyer's) red | 8-oz. container | 260 |
| (Dannon): | | |
| Extra Smooth | 4.4-oz. container | 130 |
| *Fresh Flavors* | 8-oz. container | 200 |
| (Light n' Lively) red | 8-oz. container | 230 |
| (Riché) | 6-oz. container | 180 |

| Food and Description | Measure or Quantity | Calories |
|---|---|---|
| (Sweet'N Low) | 8-oz container | 150 |
| *Yoplait:* | | |
| Regular | 6-oz. container | 190 |
| *Custard Style* | 6-oz. container | 180 |
| Strawberry: | | |
| (Breyer's) | 8-oz. container | 270 |
| (Dannon) *Fresh Flavors* | 8-oz. container | 200 |
| (Friendship) | 8-oz. container | 230 |
| (Light n' Lively) | 8-oz. container | 240 |
| *Lite-Line* (Borden) | 8-oz. container | 240 |
| (Meadow Gold) | 8-oz. container | 270 |
| (Whitney's) | 6-oz. container | 200 |
| *Yoplait,* regular | 6-oz. container | 190 |
| Strawberry-banana (Light n' Lively) | 8-oz. container | 260 |
| Strawberry colada (Colombo) | 8-oz. container | 230 |
| Tropical fruit (Sweet'N Low) | 8-oz. container | 150 |
| Vanilla: | | |
| (Breyer's) | 8-oz. container | 230 |
| (Friendship) | 8-oz. container | 210 |
| (La Yogurt) | 6-oz. container | 160 |
| (Whitney's) | 6-oz. container | 200 |
| *Yoplait, Custard Style* | 6-oz. container | 180 |
| Frozen, hard: | | |
| Banana, *Danny-in-a-Cup* | 8-oz. cup | 210 |
| Boysenberry, *Danny-On-A-Stick,* carob coated | 2½-fl.-oz. bar | 140 |
| Boysenberry swirl (Bison) | ¼ of 16-oz. container | 116 |
| Chocolate: | | |
| (Bison) | ¼ of 16-oz. container | 116 |
| (Colombo) bar, chocolate coated | 1 bar | 145 |
| (Dannon): | | |
| *Danny-in-a-Cup* | 8-fl.-oz. cup | 190 |
| *Danny-On-A-Stick,* chocolate coated | 2½-fl.-oz. bar | 130 |
| Chocolate chip (Bison) | ¼ of 16-oz. container | 116 |
| Chocolate chocolate chip (Colombo) | 4-oz. serving | 150 |
| Mocha (Colombo) bar | 1 bar | 80 |
| Piña colada: | | |
| (Colombo) | 4-oz. serving | 110 |
| (Dannon): | | |
| *(Danny-in-a-Cup* | 8-oz. cup | 210 |
| *Danny-On-A-Stick* | 2½-fl.-oz. bar | 65 |
| Raspberry, red (Dannon): | | |
| *Danny-in-a-Cup* | 8-oz. container | 210 |
| *Danny-On-A-Stick,* | | |

| Food and Description | Measure or Quantity | Calories |
|---|---|---|
| chocolate coated | 2½-fl.-oz. bar | 130 |
| Strawberry: | | |
| (Bison) | ¼ of 16-oz. container | 116 |
| (Colombo): | | |
| Regular | 4-oz. serving | 110 |
| Bar | 1 bar | 80 |
| (Dannon): | | |
| *Danny-in-a-Cup* | 8 fl. oz. | 210 |
| *Danny-Yo* | 3½ fl. oz. | 110 |
| Vanilla: | | |
| (Colombo): | | |
| Regular | 4-oz. serving | 110 |
| Bar, chocolate coated | 1 bar | 145 |
| (Dannon): | | |
| *Danny-in-a-Cup* | 8 fl. oz. | 180 |
| *Danny-On-A-Stick* | 2½-fl.-oz. bar | 65 |
| *Danny-Yo* | 3½-oz. serving | 110 |
| Frozen, soft (Colombo) | 6-fl.-oz. serving | 130 |

# Z

| Food and Description | Measure or Quantity | Calories |
|---|---|---|
| **ZINFANDEL WINE** (Louis M. Martini) regular vintage | 3 fl. oz. | 67 |
| **ZINGERS** (Dolly Madison): | | |
| Devils food | 1¼-oz. piece | 140 |
| Raspberry | 1¼-oz. piece | 130 |
| **ZITI, FROZEN:** | | |
| (Morton) Light | 11-oz. dinner | 280 |
| (Weight Watchers) | 11¼-oz. meal | 290 |
| **ZWEIBACK** (Gerber: Nabisco) | 1 piece | 30 |